WQ 18 NGW

Part 2 MRCOG:
Revision Made Easy

D0507879

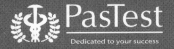

PasTest
Dedicated to your success

Dedication

This work is dedicated to: my lovely children, Sobukhosi and Nqobile for filling me with a sense of wonderful fatherhood, the Erlwanger family, Dr and Mrs Tsaurai, John Jr, Ian and Alison for all the goodwill messages during difficult times; my mother Bebi for the deep sense of love; and sisters Doras and Sipho for urging me to keep fighting.

Thank you to the following: Pretty, Emmanuel, Duduzile, Simakatso and Beata for the support over the years. I can never forget my late father Sikuba for making me a workhorse from a tender age.
SN

To my wife Veronica and our children, Ben and Meg, and to my mother Eleanor for her encouragement to study.
SL

Part 2 MRCOG: Revision Made Easy

Dr Solwayo Ngwenya MBChB, DFFP, MRCOG
Senior Registrar in Obstetrics and Gynaecology
Mpilo Central Hospital
Bulawayo
Zimbabwe

Mr Stephen Lindow MD, FCOG (SA), FRCOG
Senior Lecturer in Perinatology
Hull University
Consultant Obstetrician and Gynaecologist
Hull Royal Infirmary
Hull
UK

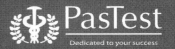

PasTest
Dedicated to your success

© 2007 PASTEST LTD

Egerton Court
Parkgate Estate
Knutsford
Cheshire
WA16 8DX

Telephone: 01565 752000

First published 2007

ISBN: 1 904627 92 7

ISBN: 978 1904627 920

A catalogue record for this book is available from the British Library.

The information contained within this book was obtained by the authors from reliable sources. However, while every effort has been made to ensure its accuracy, no responsibility for loss, damage or injury occasioned to any person acting or refraining from action as a result of information contained herein can be accepted by the publishers or authors.

PasTest Revision Books and Intensive Courses
PasTest has been established in the field of postgraduate medical education since 1972, providing revision books and intensive study courses for doctors preparing for their professional examinations.

Books and courses are available for the following specialties:
MRCGP, MRCP Parts 1 and 2, MRCPCH Parts 1 and 2, MRCPsych, MRCS, MRCOG Parts 1 and 2, DRCOG, DCH, FRCA, PLAB Parts 1 and 2.

For further details contact:
PasTest, Freepost, Knutsford, Cheshire WA16 7BR
Tel: 01565 752000 Fax: 01565 650264
www.pastest.co.uk enquiries@pastest.co.uk

Text prepared by Carnegie Book Production

Printed and bound in the UK by Athenaeum Press, Gateshead

Contents

Acknowledgements   vi

Preface   vii

Introduction   ix

Multiple Choice Questions: Questions   1
    Practice paper   3
    Gynaecology practice questions   23
    Obstetric practice questions   41

Multiple Choice Questions: Answers   59
    Answers to practice paper   61
    Answers to gynaecology practice questions   73
    Answers to obstetric practice questions   85

Essay Writing Tips   97
    Essay questions   104
    Essay answers
        Gynaecology 1–16   108
        Obstetrics 17–32   140

Objective Structured Clinical Examinations (OSCEs)   173
    Stations 1–30   175

List of abbreviations   234

Bibliography   237

Index   238

Acknowledgements

We would like to acknowledge Austin Ugwumadu, Charlotte Chaliha, Barry
Whitlow and Andrea Hermann for their contribution to the original work.
We would also like to thank Mr Davelly Mweemba MRCOG, for careful
checking of the whole manuscript for mistakes and supplying suggestions
for improvement of the work.

Preface

The MRCOG Part 2 examination remains the most difficult of all professional examinations. As postgraduate education needs candidates to seek information themselves, this book provides a good guide to preparing for this examination. At this level there are no lectures to teach and prepare candidates for the examination. A book such as this provides them with the preparation that they need. Most questions in the MRCOG Part 2 examination are clinical in nature; they demand a logical approach to tackling them. Short essays mean short essays, hence you need to be very concise in what you write. Thorough preparation, hard work, self-confidence and dedication are the key to passing this examination. This book provides a clear way of how to structure short essays, and a pool of MCQs and OSCE stations for good coverage of the MRCOG syllabus. Study very carefully how short essays are written up in flowing English with proper sentences, full stops, commas and paragraphs. Do not write lists or bullet points. This will result in a very sure fail. EMQs are not covered in this book.

Introduction

This book features:

- three MCQ papers with answers

- 32 short essays covering both obstetrics and gynaecology

- 30 OSCE questions equivalent, to three practice exams.

The current structure of the MRCOG Part 2 examination consists of a written part and a clinical exam (OSCE). The written paper consists of:

- 225 MCQs lasting 1 hour and 30 minutes

- short essays divided into:

  - paper 1: four obstetrics questions lasting for 1 hour and 45 minutes

  - paper 2: four gynaecology questions lasting for 1 hour and 45 minutes

- 40 EMQs lasting for 1 hour.

Only those candidates who pass the written paper go for the OSCEs. The syllabus for the MRCOG Part 2 examination, as published by the Royal College of Obstetricians and Gynaecologists, is now summarised.

Genetics and embryology

Comprehensive knowledge of normal and abnormal karyotypes, the inheritance of genetic disorders, the genetic causes of infertility and early abortion, as well as the ability to transmit this knowledge to patients, are necessary to discuss their implications as well as any ethical dilemmas.

Anatomy

Continuing comprehensive knowledge of anatomy is needed, particularly as applied to surgical procedures undertaken by the obstetrician and gynaecologist.

Pathology, biochemistry and endocrinology

Thorough knowledge of the pathology of the genital tract and associated structures and sound understanding of biochemistry of mother and fetus are necessary, together with in-depth knowledge of metabolism. Although endocrinological knowledge of all organs is required, extensive knowledge is expected of the endocrine organs as applied to reproductive medicine.

Pharmacology

Comprehensive knowledge of all aspects of pharmacology is required with particular knowledge of those drugs that will be used in obstetrics and gynaecology.

Immunology

Candidates are expected to understand basic immunology and how this may be changed in pregnancy, and fetal development of the immune system, with particular knowledge of rhesus and other isoimmunisations.

Infectious diseases

Candidates must have comprehensive knowledge of the infectious diseases affecting pregnant and non-pregnant women as well as the fetus in utero, plus knowledge of epidemiology, diagnostic techniques, prophylaxis, immunisation, and use of antibiotics and antiviral agents.

Epidemiology and statistics

Candidates should understand how to apply statistical analysis, to collect data, to have knowledge of setting up clinical trials and the ability to interpret data.

Normal pregnancy

Candidates must have knowledge of all maternal and fetal systems, and comprehensive knowledge of antepartum care, its aims and method of implementation. Similarly, they should have knowledge of intra partum care, which should include in-depth knowledge of obstetric analgesia and anaesthesia.

Abnormal pregnancy

Candidates are expected to have clear knowledge of all aspects of abnormality in pregnancy, labour and the puerperium, together with their management. Detailed knowledge of neonatal resuscitation is mandatory.

Pre-pregnancy and post-pregnancy counselling

Candidates should demonstrate their ability to advise patients about any aspect of obstetric or gynaecological disease.

Maternal and perinatal mortality

Candidates are expected to be familiar with definitions and concepts, as well as to be conversant with confidential enquiries into maternal deaths and the reports on birth surveys.

Gynaecology

Candidates should exhibit proficiency in history taking, in general, and gynaecology, in particular, and at general and gynaecological examination. Detailed knowledge of all basic gynaecological procedures, as well as the ability to perform more common gynaecological operations, are required. Candidates will be expected to have a knowledge of more complicated procedures, eg in oncology, although at the level of the membership examination proficiency in these areas will not be expected.

Prepubertal gynaecology

Candidates should have thorough knowledge of normal and abnormal sexual development, paediatric pathology and its management, and normal puberty and its disorders.

Disorders of menstruation

Based on the physiology of normal menstruation, candidates should have in-depth understanding of the pathophysiology of menstrual disorders, their investigation and management, and the menopause.

Infertility

Candidates should know about causes, investigation and management of infertility, together with basic knowledge in the techniques involved in in vitro fertilisation.

Contraception and abortion

All methods of contraception should be thoroughly understood and candidates are obliged to present evidence of practical experience. The reasons for, techniques and complications of, performing therapeutic abortion should be understood.

Psychosexual medicine

A thorough understanding of the principles of psychosexual medicine is required.

Gynaecological oncology

Candidates should understand the epidemiology and aetiology of gynaecological tumours. The principles of carcinogenesis, tumour immunology and pathology, together with diagnostic techniques and staging of gynaecological tumours, are essential. They should also have knowledge about basic principles of treatment – surgery, radiotherapy and chemotherapy – together with knowledge of terminal care from gynaecological malignancy.

Multiple Choice
Questions: Questions

PRACTICE PAPER

225 questions: time allowed 1 hour, 45 mins
Indicate your answers with T (true) or F (false) in the boxes provided.

With regard to recurrent vulvovaginal candiasis:

1   It is defined as one attack every year

2   It affects 15% of healthy women of reproductive age

3   It may be found in AIDS patients

4   It is caused only by *Candida albicans*

5   It responds well to single course treatments

With regard to emergency contraception:

6   It must be given within 72 hours of unprotected intercourse

7   The Mirena coil can be used

8   Levonorgestrel is the drug of choice

9   The combined oral contraceptive pill (COCP) can be used

10   A copper IUCD (intrauterine contraceptive device) can be used up to 5 days after the earliest calculated date of ovulation or 5 days after the first act of unprotected coitus

PRACTICE PAPER QUESTIONS

Answers on pages 61–71

Complications of assisted reproduction are:

11   Ovarian hyperstimulation syndrome

12   Ovarian cancer

13   Ectopic pregnancy

14   Diabetes mellitus

15   Endometrial cancer

Factors that increase the risk of failed termination of pregnancy include:

16   Nulliparity

17   Termination at less than 6 weeks' gestation

18   Acute retroversion of the uterus

19   Uterine abnormalities

20   Uterine fibroids

With regard to emergency contraception:

21   The copper IUCD should not be fitted more than 5 days after the first act of unprotected intercourse

22   The copper IUCD has spermicidal activity

23   The copper IUCD prevents implantation

24   The copper IUCD is less effective than the levonorgestrel-only method

25   The copper IUCD is contraindicated in a nulliparous woman

With regard to the use of progesterone-only emergency contraception:

26 The overall pregnancy rate after use is $< 0.5\%$

27 It can be used only once during one cycle

28 It is contraindicated in a woman with a past history of an ectopic pregnancy

29 It is contraindicated in patients with a history of deep vein thrombosis

With regard to urinary tract infections:

30 They are strongly associated with the use of diaphragms

31 They are more common in secretors of histoblood group antigens

32 *Escherichia coli* is the most common community-acquired pathogen

33 They are reported in 5% of girls aged up to 1 year

34 In school-aged children, it is more common in girls than in boys

The following are normal parameters of bladder function:

35 Residual urine < 100 ml

36 A peak flow rate on voiding of more than 25 ml/s for a voided volume of 150 ml

37 A detrusor pressure rise on voiding of > 50 cmH$_2$O

38 A detrusor pressure rise of < 15 cmH$_2$O on filling the bladder to 500 ml

39 First desire to void at > 400 ml

With regard to detrusor overactivity:

40 Cystoscopy is a useful diagnostic tool

41 Patients have an increased bladder wall thickness compared with those with urodynamic stress incontinence

42 Most cases in women are the result of bladder-neck obstruction

43 There is a good relationship between symptoms and urodynamic findings

44 It is seen more commonly in those with neurotic personality traits

Risk factors for ectopic pregnancy include:

45 Smoking

46 Salpingitis isthmica nodosa

47 Diethylstilbestrol

48 Luteal phase defects

Causes of primary amenorrhoea in a girl with normal external genitalia include:

49 Kallmann's syndrome

50 Turner's syndrome

51 Congenital adrenal hyperplasia

52 Craniopharyngioma

In gestational trophoblastic disease:

53 Complete moles are usually androgenic in origin

54 Partial moles are usually triploid

55 Partial moles do not transform into choriocarcinomas

56 An embryo is usually present with a partial mole

57 Heterozygous complete moles are more common than homozygous ones

With regard to intraoperative complications:

58 The risk of bowel injury at laparoscopic surgery is 1%

59 Bowel damage during laparoscopy more commonly involves the small bowel

60 Non-absorbable sutures should be used to repair bladder perforations

61 Insertion of a Verress needle into the bladder requires catheterisation for 5–7 days

62 The risk of ureteric injury is lowest in laparoscopic versus vaginal and abdominal surgery

With regard to the following contraceptive methods:

63 After stopping the combined pill, 60% of women will ovulate by their third cycle

64 5% of women will be amenorrhoeic 6 months after stopping the combined pill

65 Following the final injection of depot medroxyprogesterone, ovulation returns after 4–5 months

66 Women with a low body mass index (BMI) are at increased risk of 'post-pill' amenorrhoea

The clinical staging of cervical cancer includes:

67   Cystoscopy

68   Proctoscopy

69   Laparoscopy

70   Chest radiograph

71   Cervical biopsy

In invasive carcinoma of the cervix:

72   In stage IB tumours, size has little relevance to the 5-year survival rate

73   In stage IIB disease, there is extension of tumour from the cervix into the lower third of the vagina

74   Barrel-shaped endocervical lesions have a worse prognosis than cervical cancers of a similar stage

75   Stage for stage, adenocarcinoma of the cervix has a poorer survival rate than squamous lesions

76   Pelvic exenteration is contraindicated if there is a central recurrence after radiotherapy

In ovarian cancer:

77 Thirty per cent of women have metastasis by the time of presentation

78 Mucinous and endometrioid carcinomas are more likely to be associated with an earlier stage and lower grade than serous cystadenocarcinomas

79 The tumour marker CA-125 is associated only with mucinous tumours

80 The histological type, rather than clinical extent of the tumour, is more important in determining prognosis

81 Pleural effusion indicates a stage IV disease

Bacterial vaginosis:

82 Is more common in white than in black women

83 Is not seen in virgins or lesbians

84 Shows clue cells

85 Shows a pH of vaginal discharge of < 4.5

86 Is the most common cause of vaginal discharge in women of childbearing age

In gonorrhoea:

87   Fifty per cent of women with gonorrhoea have concomitant chlamydial infection

88   The incubation period is between 2 and 3 months

89   *Neisseria gonorrhoeae*, the cause, is a Gram-positive diplococcus

90   Diagnosis can be made on the presence of positive serology

91   At least 50% of infected women are asymptomatic

Risk factors associated with increasing the need for chemotherapy after evacuation of a hydatidiform mole are:

92   Younger age

93   Pre-evacuation hCG > 100 000 IU/L

94   Gestational age > uterine size

95   Use of oral contraceptives before evacuation

96   Bilateral cystic ovarian enlargement

With regard to endometrioid carcinoma of the ovary:

97   It accounts for 10% of all ovarian tumours

98   Borderline variants have a good prognosis

99   Fifteen per cent are associated with endometrial carcinoma

100   Twenty per cent are seen in continuity with recognisable endometriosis

With regard to borderline tumours of the ovary:

101   Ten per cent of all epithelial tumours are borderline

102   They are most commonly serous in type

103   DNA-ploidy is the most important prognostic factor

104   The 5-year survival rate for mucinous borderline tumours is better than for serous tumours

105   Most are confined to the ovary

Uterine leiomyosarcoma:

106   Is the most common sarcoma of the uterus

107   Arises from a fibroid in 20% of cases

108   Occurs mainly in nulliparous patients

109   Is more common in Afro–Caribbean women

110   Occurs in 20% of cases with vascular invasion at the time of presentation

HIV infection:

111   Is common in heterosexuals

112   Affects more women than men

The following are 'soft' markers for aneuploidy:

113   Hyperechogenic bowel

114   Hypoplastic left heart

115   Choroid plexus cyst

116   Cardiac echogenic foci

117   Fetal pelvicalyceal dilatation

With regard to heart disease in pregnancy:

118   Eisenmenger's syndrome is a contraindication to pregnancy

119   During pregnancy, plasma volume starts to increase as early as 6 weeks

120   In high-risk cases termination of pregnancy should be offered

121   There is a risk of intrauterine growth retardation (IUGR)

122   Delivery should be by Caesarean section

Tocolysis:

123   Should be given in antepartum haemorrhage

124   Can be given as atosiban, which is as effective as ritodrine in stopping preterm labour

125   Allows administration of steroids and in utero transfer

126   Must be given for 72 hours

127   Improves perinatal death rates

Group B streptococcal infection:

128 Is caused by a Gram-negative bacterium

129 Can colonise the rectum or vagina in 28% of pregnant women

130 In neonates can be reduced by intravenous antibiotics during labour

With regard to haemoglobinopathies in pregnancy:

131 Sickle cell disease is common in white women

132 There is a risk of miscarriage

133 Thalassaemia major carries a risk of thromboembolism

134 Both sickle cell disease and thalassaemia major carry a risk of maternal infection

Dyspareunia after childbirth:

135 Can be from physical or psychological causes

136 Can be associated with anxiety and depression

137 Is always secondary to a physical cause

Congenital cleft lip and palate:

138 Is more common as a unilateral than a bilateral defect

139 Is not associated with aneuploidy

140 Has increased risk in future pregnancies

141 Is associated with antiepileptic medications

With regard to systemic lupus erythematosus (SLE) in pregnancy:

142   There is a decreased risk of flare-up in pregnancy

143   It is associated with an increased risk of abortion

144   Anti-Ro antibodies are present in 15% of patients

145   Anti-Ro antibodies cross the placenta

146   Cutaneous lupus is seen in 50% of babies of anti-Ro-positive mothers

With regard to rheumatoid arthritis in pregnancy:

147   The disease will deteriorate in most women during pregnancy

148   Symptoms usually improve post partum

149   There is an increased rate of miscarriage

150   Azathioprine is contraindicated

151   Sulfasalazine is safe in pregnancy

Peripartum cardiomyopathy:

152   Can occur up to 6 months post partum

153   Is more common in primiparous patients

154   Is more common in black women

155   Requires anticoagulation

156   Is commonly recurrent

The normal haemodynamic changes in pregnancy include:

157   An increase in plasma volume, particularly during the third trimester

158   A decrease in pulse volume

159   A return to normal of the rise in cardiac output in pregnancy in the first 24 hours post partum

160   A diastolic murmur, which is a common, normal physiological finding

In the management of labour:

161   Engagement of the vertex occurs when the biparietal diameter passes the pelvic outlet

162   Active management of labour reduces the risk of Caesarean section

163   Oxytocin should not be used if cephalopelvic disproportion is suspected

164   Amniotomy is associated with an increased risk of instrumental delivery

165   Most women who have had a previous Caesarean section for cephalopelvic disproportion will have a subsequent vaginal delivery

Anti-D prophylaxis:

166 Should be given to all non-sensitised rhesus (Rh) D-negative women after amniocentesis or chorionic villus sampling (CVS)

167 Should be given to all non-sensitised Rh D-negative women after a threatened miscarriage

168 Can be sensitised by undetected fetomaternal haemorrhage in the third trimester in 90% of cases

169 Should be routinely administered (500 IU anti-D) to all non-sensitised Rh-negative primigravidas at 28 weeks' and 34 weeks' gestation

170 In a woman who has any sensitising event after 20 weeks' gestation should be followed by Kleihauer testing

In a woman with prosthetic heart valves:

171 There is a high risk of bacterial endocarditis during delivery

172 Usually there is a decreased cardiac reserve

173 Heparin use for anticoagulation is associated with a higher rate of thromboembolic complications

174 Oxytocin is contraindicated in labour

175 The risk of teratogenicity from warfarin is greatest at 9–12 weeks' gestation

With regard to the small-for-gestational-age (SGA) fetus:

176　An amniotic fluid index < 0.5 cm is associated with an increased risk of an Apgar score < 7 at 5 minutes

177　Of fetuses with an abdominal circumference and estimated fetal weight < fifth centile, 70% have chromosomal defects

178　Of normally formed stillbirths, 20% are SGA

179　The ratio of head to abdominal circumference is more accurate than abdominal circumference or estimated fetal weight (EFW) alone in predicting the SGA fetus

180　It is associated with the development of type 2 diabetes in adult life

With regard to chickenpox in pregnancy:

181　The incubation period is 5–10 days

182　Shingles before 20 weeks' gestation has a 1% risk of fetal abnormality

183　Varicella immunoglobulin given to the mother within the first 24 hours of contact with chickenpox prevents intrauterine infection

184　Congenital varicella may be detected on a second trimester anomaly scan

With regard to amniotic fluid:

185   The 15th and 95th centiles for the amniotic fluid index are 5–15 cm

186   It is reduced in upper gastrointestinal obstruction

187   It is reduced in bilateral uropathy

188   It is reduced in fetuses with neural tube defects

189   It is increased in maternal diabetes

In fetal red cell alloimmunisation:

190   The indirect Coombs' test can detect the presence of antibodies in serum

191   Maternal serum anti-D < 4 IU/ml is not associated with severe fetal anaemia

192   There is an increase in Doppler blood flow velocity in fetal vessels in severe anaemia

193   Severe fetal anaemia is always characterised by poor fetal movements and hydrops

194   The survival rate of a hydropic fetus after intrauterine transfusion is about 50%

With regard to postpartum haemorrhage:

195   It may be associated with platelet deficiency

196   Fresh-frozen plasma (FFP) should ideally be given with every 2
      units of blood

197   Hyperkalaemia may be a complication of blood transfusion

198   The blood volume should be restored until the central venous
      pressure (CVP) is 5 cmH$_2$O

199   Cryoprecipitate should be given if the fibrinogen level is
      < 1.0 g/dl

Herpes gestationis in pregnancy:

200   Is caused by a herpes virus

201   Is spread by droplets

202   Is diagnosed on the serology results

203   Usually recurs in subsequent pregnancies

204   Is associated with low birthweight and preterm delivery

205   Means that systemic steroids should be withheld until after
      delivery

In HIV in pregnancy:

206   Without intervention the mother-to-child transmission (MCT) rate is up to 30%

207   Breast-feeding doubles the risk of CT

208   There is an increased risk of complications at caesarean section

209   A viral load < 2000 copies/ml is not associated with fetal infection

210   Antiretroviral treatment should be commenced as soon as the diagnosis is known

With regard to the death of one twin in a monochorionic twin pregnancy:

211   It is associated with a 25% risk of death in the surviving twin

212   It is associated with a 50% risk of cerebral damage in the surviving twin

213   The appearance of porencephaly in the surviving twin indicates severe brain damage

214   Delivery should be delayed as long as possible until there is structural evidence of brain damage

215   Delivery should be by Caesarean section

216   There is no risk of fetal brain damage in the surviving twin of a dichorionic twin pregnancy

In any set of observations:

217   The mean is less than the mode

218   Half the observations are less than the median

219   If the data are skewed to the right, the median is less than the mean

220   The mode is always the most frequently occurring value

221   The variance is the square root of the standard deviation

Urine cytology was studied in 100 women with haematuria to assess the accuracy of urine cytology in the detection of bladder cancer. In this group, 20 women had positive cytology. At the end of the study ten women had confirmed bladder cancers, but only five had positive cytology. With regard to urine cytology for the detection of bladder cancer:

222   The sensitivity of the test is 50%

223   The specificity of the test is 10%

224   The negative predictive value is 5%

225   The positive predictive value is 25%

PRACTICE PAPER QUESTIONS

GYNAECOLOGY PRACTICE QUESTIONS

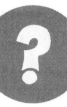

Indicate your answers with T (true) or F (false) in the boxes provided.

With regard to cervical screening:

1   The screening programme targets women aged between 20 and 50 years

2   Pap smear tests have a false-negative rate of 15–25%

3   The incidence of mild dyskaryosis is approximately 10%

4   The incidence of moderate dyskaryosis is 5%

5   The incidence of severe dyskaryosis is 0.5%

Risk factors for anal sphincter injury are:

6   Midline episiotomy

7   Prolonged second stage of labour

8   Fetal macrosomia

9   Occipitoposterior position

10   Elective Caesarean section

Answers on page 73–84

Faecal incontinence

11   Is more common in women than in men

12   Occurs in 1% of women after vaginal delivery

13   Increases with age

14   Has the most significant aetiological factor after childbirth of pudendal neuropathy

In a woman with a history of a previous third-degree tear, the risk of faecal incontinence after another vaginal delivery:

15   Is reduced by elective episiotomy

16   Is related to the degree of pudendal neuropathy

17   Is increased if the woman is symptomatic

18   Is reduced by perineal massage

In a woman with a history of stress incontinence:

19   α-Agonists have been shown to reduce the number of stress incontinence episodes

20   Conservative treatment achieves long-term cure in most

21   Electrical stimulation acts by stimulating the autonomic nervous supply

22   Oestrogen therapy has been shown to reduce symptoms

With regard to the surgical management of stress incontinence:

23 An anterior repair will correct incontinence as well as a coexisting cystocele

24 The tension-free vaginal tape procedure has a similar success rate to Burch colposuspension

25 The Marshall–Martchetti–Krantz and Burch colposuspension procedures will correct a coexisting cystocele

26 A Burch colposuspension will worsen a coexisting rectocele or enterocele

27 Needle suspension procedures have a long-term success rate of about 50–60%

With regard to premature ovarian failure:

28 The incidence is about 5%

29 It occurs in 50% of patients presenting with secondary amenorrhoea

30 Hot flushes occur in about 50% of patients

31 Symptoms are related to the levels of LH (luteinising hormone) and FSH (follicle-stimulating hormone)

GYNAECOLOGY QUESTIONS

With regard to azoospermia:

32   Two-thirds of cases are caused by genital tract obstruction

33   Obstructive azoospermia is seen in about 50% of men with cystic fibrosis

34   Testicular biopsy samples show reduced spermatogenesis in obstructive spermatogenesis

35   Karyotyping is always recommended in cases of azoospermia

36   It is seen in 30% of infertile men

In cases involving ovarian accidents:

37   Among surgically managed cases, the frequency of malignant tumours is about 45% in premenopausal women and about 13% in postmenopausal women

38   About 25% of cases of torsion occur in children

39   Cystadenomas are the most common tumours leading to torsion

40   Around 15% of ovarian torsions involve ovarian malignancy

In cases of haemorrhage into or from ovarian cysts:

41   Rupture occurs most commonly on days 3–5 of the menstrual cycle

42   Two-thirds of cases involve the right ovary

43   The risk is increased by anticoagulants despite normal coagulation indices

44   It may cause haemolytic jaundice

Factors that increase the risk of ovarian hyperstimulation syndrome include:

45 Older age

46 A higher number of mature and immature follicles

47 Use of hCG (human chorionic gonadotrophin) for luteal support

48 Pregnancy

49 Higher body mass index (BMI)

With regard to assisted reproduction:

50 Multiple pregnancy is more common with superovulation with/ without intrauterine insemination (IUI) than in vitro fertilisation (IVF)/intracytoplasmic sperm injection (ICSI) cycles

51 There is a higher risk of infants of low birthweight

52 The heterotopic pregnancy rate is about 5% in IVF pregnancies

53 The ectopic pregnancy rate is about 15%

The following statements about clomifene citrate are correct:

54 The ovulation rate in a normally oestrogenised woman is about 50%

55 The pregnancy rate is 30–40%

56 Side effects are dose dependent

57 The use of clomifene citrate results in a 20% increase in endogenous follicle-stimulating hormone (FSH) and luteinising hormone (LH) concentrations

Gonadotrophin-releasing hormone (GnRH) analogues:

58   Are synthesised by substitution of amino acids at positions 4 and 8 of the decapeptide GnRH

59   Lead to a higher rate of ovulation and conception than gonadotrophin regimens

60   Result in most women being hypo-oestrogenic within a week

61   Can cause a reduction in bone density, which is reversible after stopping treatment

Biochemical changes seen in congenital adrenal hyperplasia as a result of 21-hydroxylase deficiency include:

62   Increased urinary ketosteroids

63   Increased serum aldosterone

64   Decreased serum testosterone

65   Increased serum 17-hydroxyprogesterone

The following metabolic changes are seen after the menopause:

66   A rise in plasma testosterone

67   A rise in plasma calcium

68   A decrease in plasma androstenedione

69   A decrease in plasma cholesterol

The following are seen in association with Turner's syndrome:

70   Lymphoedema

71   Hypogonadotrophic hypogonadism

72   A single Barr body

73   Increased incidence with maternal age

74   Horseshoe kidney

Hyperprolactinaemia:

75   Occurs in 25% of patients with hyperthyroidism

76   Occurs in 25% of patients with acromegaly

77   May be associated with renal failure

78   Is a side effect of metoclopramide use

79   Has pituitary causes mainly as a result of prolactin-secreting microadenomas

Recurrent miscarriage:

80   Is associated with diabetes

81   Is increased in women with hyperthyroidism

82   Is a result of antiphospholipid antibodies in about 15% of women

83   When caused by parental chromosomal abnormality, Robertsonian translocations are the most frequently identified

84   In women with antiphospholipid syndrome, results in an 85–90% risk of miscarriage without treatment

GYNAECOLOGY QUESTIONS

Precocious puberty:

85   Is defined as the onset of puberty before 8 years of age in girls

86   May be a feature of neurofibromatosis

87   May be caused by Cushing's disease

88   May be caused by hyperthyroidism

89   Reveals elevated basal gonadotrophin levels in the true form

In women with hirsutism:

90   Total serum testosterone levels are usually raised

91   Serum testosterone levels correlate well with the severity of hirsutism

92   Circulating dehydroepiandrosterone (sulphate or DHEAS) level is usually raised

93   Polycystic ovarian syndrome is the most common cause

94   Most androgen-secreting tumours are benign

With regard to the progesterone-only pill:

95   Fifty per cent of women will continue to ovulate

96   Follicular development is inhibited in only 10–20% of women

97   The half-life is approximately 8 hours

98   The failure rate is higher in those with a low BMI

99   It is associated with an increased number of functional ovarian cysts

Risk factors for osteoporosis include:

100 Early menopause

101 Hypothyroidism

102 Cigarette smoking

103 Type 1 diabetes

104 Hypergonadism

The following drugs are associated with hyperprolactinaemia:

105 Haloperidol

106 Prochlorperazine

107 Bromocriptine

108 Methyldopa

109 Cimetidine

Plasma gonadotrophin levels are increased in:

110 Turner's syndrome

111 Kallmann's syndrome

112 Testicular feminisation syndrome

113 McCune–Albright syndrome

114 Anorexia nervosa

GYNAECOLOGY QUESTIONS

In cervical intraepithelial neoplasia (CIN):

115 Over 99% of cases contain human papillomavirus (HPV)

116 HPV subtypes 12 and 14 are high risk for CIN

117 Of CIN3 lesions 60% progress to cancer within 10 years

118 HPV is a non-enveloped RNA virus

119 Regions E3 and E4 code for oncoproteins

Risk factors for cervical cancer and CIN include:

120 Nulliparity

121 Cigarette smoking

122 Previous CIN

123 Presence of other genital tract neoplasia

124 High alcohol intake

With regard to CIN:

125 It usually affects the epithelium but not the gland crypts

126 In CIN3 the mean depth of crypt involvement is > 5 mm

127 Nuclear abnormalities are the most important feature in assessing severity

In cervical adenocarcinoma in situ/cervical glandular intraepithelial neoplasia (CGIN):

128   There are no specific colposcopic features

129   Of patients 75% show a glandular abnormality on cytology

130   In a third of cases there is an invasive squamous lesion or CIN

131   The majority of cases lie in the transformation zone

132   Isolated adenocarcinoma in situ (AIS) high in the endocervical canal is uncommon in young women

In vaginal intraepithelial neoplasia (VIN):

133   Ten per cent of women are under 40 years of age

134   Over 50% of patients are asymptomatic

135   The recurrence rate may be as high as 40%

In endometrial hyperplasia:

136   Atypical hyperplasia is the only form with a significant risk of progression to malignancy

137   A coexistent carcinoma may be found in 5–10% of patients with atypical hyperplasia

138   Risk of progression of cystic hyperplasia is < 5%

139   Cystic hyperplasia may be managed on the basis of recurrent symptoms

With regard to vulval cancer:

140 The majority of cases are squamous cell

141 The risk of progression of VIN to vulval cancer is 25%

142 The risk of progression of VIN is higher in multifocal compared with unifocal disease

143 Paget's disease is associated with concomitant genital tract malignancy in 40% of cases

144 The risk of malignant transformation of lichen sclerosus is 10%

With regard to the treatment of vulval cancer:

145 Stage II lesions have a high risk of groin node metastasis

146 Lateralised type 1 and 2 tumours rarely involve groin nodes

147 Stage I lateralised lesions should be treated with radical vulvectomy and bilateral lymphadenectomy

148 The groin nodes should always be removed

149 Younger women have a higher incidence of nodal disease

Features associated with intrauterine exposure to diethylstilbestrol are:

150 Cervical cockscomb

151 Vaginal adenosis

152 Clear-cell adenocarcinoma

153 CIN

Krukenberg's tumours:

154   Occur via coelomic spread

155   Are sarcomas

156   Secrete oestrogen

157   Secrete gastrin

158   Contain signet cells

Which of the following statements about chemotherapy is/are true:

159   Doxorubicin (Adriamycin) causes cardiac myopathy

160   Methotrexate causes haemorrhagic cystitis

161   Vincristine causes peripheral neuropathy

162   Cisplatin causes ototoxity

The following tumours are of germ-cell origin:

163   Yolk sac tumour

164   Brenner's tumour

165   Endometrioid tumour

166   Embryonal cell tumour

167   Teratoma

GYNAECOLOGY QUESTIONS

Serous cystadenocarcinoma:

168   Is the most common malignant ovarian tumour

169   Often contains psammoma bodies

170   Is bilateral in less than 20% of cases

171   Presents as stage III disease in 50% of cases

With regard to 5α-reductase deficiency:

172   It occurs as a result of a mutation in the short arm of the Y chromosome

173   It is associated with virilisation at puberty

174   Testosterone production occurs normally in the testes

175   Anti-Müllerian hormone production is deficient

176   Affected individuals have ambiguous genitalia

The following reduce(s) the risk of wound dehiscence:

177   Tension sutures

178   Mass closure technique

179   Prophylactic antibiotics

180   Polyglycolic sutures

The ureter:

181   Is retroperitoneal in its abdominal course

182   Passes along the posterior medial aspect of psoas major

183   Is crossed inferiorly by the uterine artery

184   Enters the bladder at the dome

185   Is crossed by ovarian vessels

With regard to innervation of the bladder and the urethra:

186   The main supply is sympathetic

187   Cell bodies of the sympathetic supply arise from S2–S4

188   The parasympathetic supply originates from T10–L2

189   Parasympathetic effects are mediated by α-receptors and β-receptors

190   Pelvic splanchnic nerves supply the rhabdosphincter

With regard to peritoneal closure:

191   Non-closure of the peritoneum is associated with increased febrile morbidity

192   Peritoneal closure at Caesarean section increases the risk of bladder adhesions

193   Closure of the peritoneum after vaginal surgery is recommended

194   The need for postoperative analgesia is reduced if the peritoneum is not closed

195   Non-closure of the peritoneum is associated with a quicker return of bowel activity

With regard to a simple unilateral ovarian cyst < 5 cm in diameter with a normal carcinoembryonic antigen (CA)-125 in a postmenopausal woman:

196   It can be managed conservatively

197   Gives a risk of malignancy of about 10%

198   Cytological examination of aspirated cyst fluid is a useful test

199   Fifty per cent resolve spontaneously within 3 months

In cases of ectopic pregnancy:

200   In the confidential enquiry into maternal deaths ectopic pregnancy remains a major cause of death in the first trimester

201   A β-hCG rise of 66% in 48 hours suggests an ectopic pregnancy rather than an intrauterine pregnancy

202   The serum progesterone level gives good differentiation between intrauterine and ectopic pregnancies

203   Diagnostic laparoscopy has a false-positive rate of 5%

204   A serum progesterone value > 25 ng/ml suggests an ectopic pregnancy

With regard to endometriosis:

205   The incidence has a peak prevalence between 20 and 35 years of age

206   The risk is increased sevenfold if there is an affected first-degree relative

207   It is more common in dizygotic than monozygotic twins

208   The most common presenting symptom is pelvic pain

209   Dyspareunia is reported in over 50% of cases

Side effects of danazol include:

210   Acne

211   Cholestatic jaundice

212   Hirsutism

213   Irreversible deepening of the voice

214   Thrombocytopenia

Gestrinone:

215   Acts via binding to progesterone receptors

216   Exerts anti-oestrogenic activity via binding to oestrogen receptors

217   Has no effect on basal gonadotrophin levels

218   Causes amenorrhoea within 3 months in 70% of patients

219   Reduces sex hormone-binding globulin levels

Risk factors for endometrial carcinoma include:

220   Early menopause

221   Obesity

222   Nulliparity

223   Smoking

224   COCP

225   Progesterone-only pill

Indicate your answers with T (true) or F (false) in the boxes provided.

With regard to obstetric cholestasis:

1 Family studies suggest an autosomal recessive mode of inheritance

2 The risk of stillbirth is related to deterioration in serum transaminase levels

3 Doppler studies have been shown to be useful in predicting fetal risk

4 Ursodeoxycholic acid use is associated with an improvement in total bile acids and liver enzymes

Pathological adherence of the placenta is associated with:

5 Bicornuate uterus

6 Fetal distress in labour

7 Placenta praevia

8 Previous Caesarean section

9 Submucosal myomas

Answers on page 85–96

Fetal alcohol syndrome is associated with:

10   Chromosomal abnormalities

11   Epicanthic folds

12   Spina bifida

13   Macrosomia

14   Renal abnormalities

Idiopathic thrombocytopenic purpura (ITP):

15   Is commonly complicated by postpartum haemorrhage

16   Is associated with an increased risk of perinatal mortality

17   Is confirmed by increased numbers of metamyelocytes in the bone marrow

18   Is an autoimmune disease

The following vessels carry oxygenated blood in the fetus:

19   Umbilical artery

20   Ductus venosus

21   Inferior vena cava as it enters the right atrium

22   Carotid artery

23   Umbilical vein

A raised maternal serum α-fetoprotein (AFP) level at 16 weeks' gestation may be associated with:

24   Threatened abortion

25   Aneuploidy

26   Molar pregnancy

27   Turner's syndrome

28   Down's syndrome

Routine second-trimester anomaly scanning in the UK:

29   Detects most cases of neural tube defects

30   Detects most cases of congenital heart defects

31   Detects most cases of trisomy 21

32   Detects most cases of cerebral palsy

33   Detects most cases of major renal abnormality

Neonatal jaundice is associated with:

34   Galactosaemia

35   Sickle cell disease

36   Blood group incompatibility

37   Hypothyroidism

38   Phenylketonuria

OBSTETRIC QUESTIONS

Cytomegalovirus (CMV) in pregnancy:

39 May be acquired from only primary (not secondary) maternal infection

40 May always be present in the fetus within the first 24 hours of birth

41 Gives the highest risk of transmission to the fetus when infection occurs during the second trimester

42 Is more common in lower socioeconomic groups

43 Is the most common congenital infection in the UK

Face presentation:

44 Occurs in 1:500 births

45 Is more favourable for vaginal delivery in the mentoposterior than the mentoanterior position

46 Presents the submentobregmatic diameter to the pelvic brim

47 Is associated with anencephaly

48 Is associated with prematurity

OBSTETRIC QUESTIONS

With regard to iron supplementation in pregnancy:

49   In women with a healthy diet, routine iron supplementation improves pregnancy outcome

50   Ferrous sulphate results in fewer gastrointestinal complications than ferrous gluconate

51   Parenteral iron causes the same haematological response as oral iron

52   A higher haemoglobin level reduces the risk of postpartum haemorrhage

53   It reduces the risk of antepartum haemorrhage

The following disorders are correctly associated with mode of inheritance:

54   Congenital adrenal hyperplasia – autosomal dominant

55   Tuberous sclerosis – autosomal dominant

56   Marfan's syndrome – autosomal recessive

57   Gaucher's disease – autosomal recessive

58   Familial hypercholesterolaemia – autosomal recessive

The normal electrocardiogram (ECG) in pregnancy shows:

59   A loud, third heart sound

60   A Q wave in lead III

61   A longer P–R interval

62   An increase in heart rate

OBSTETRIC QUESTIONS

With regard to fetal neural tube defects:

63   The cerebellum is affected in 50% of cases

64   The level of the lesion predicts outcome

65   A raised acetylcholinesterase level in amniotic fluid is diagnostic

66   Limb movement is a good prognostic sign of limb function after delivery

67   It may be associated with hydrocephalus

With regard to biophysical assessment of the fetus:

68   An SGA fetus has smaller heart rate accelerations compared with a normal-sized fetus of comparable age

69   Fetal breathing is decreased by maternal caffeine intake

70   At 40 weeks' gestation a normal fetus will spend 28% of its time breathing when it is active

71   A biophysical profile is a good assessment of fetal compromise in cases of maternal diabetes

72   Fetal breathing movements increase just before delivery

With regard to umbilical artery Doppler scanning:

73   It reduces the incidence of emergency Caesarean sections in high-risk pregnancies

74   It is dependent on the angle of insonation

75   The resistance index of 0 occurs when the end-diastolic velocities are absent or reversed

76   It is dimensionless

With regard to thyroid disease in pregnancy:

77   Hyperthyroidism occurs in 25% of pregnant women

78   Hypothyroidism occurs in < 1% of pregnancies

79   Thyroid peroxidase antibodies are associated with hypothyroidism

80   Thyrotrophin receptor-stimulating antibodies are a risk factor for Graves' disease

81   Thyroid peroxidase antibodies in early pregnancy are associated with a 20% chance of postpartum thyroid dysfunction

Transvaginal ultrasound measurements of cervical length in pregnancy are indicated for:

82   Previous spontaneous vaginal delivery at 14–28 weeks' gestation

83   Previous first-trimester miscarriage

84   Previous LLETZ (large loop excision of the transformation zone) or cone biopsy for an abnormal smear

85   All multiple pregnancies

86   Maternal request

OBSTETRIC QUESTIONS

The following hormones in the fetal circulation are predominantly of maternal origin:

87   Oestrogen

88   Progesterone

89   Insulin

90   Adrenocorticotrophic hormone (ACTH)

91   Thyroid-stimulating hormone (TSH)

With regard to obstetric fistulas:

92   Rectovaginal fistulas are more common than vesicovaginal fistulas

93   They usually present the day after delivery

94   The methylene blue test may distinguish a small bladder fistula from a ureteric fistula

95   Repair should be performed immediately during the postpartum period

96   The suprapubic route of repair should be used because it has a better success rate than the vaginal route

Shoulder dystocia:

97   Occurs in 1 in 1000 deliveries

98   Occurs when the bisacromial diameter is greater than the diameter of the pelvic outlet

99   Is associated with a long second stage of labour

100   Has a risk of recurrence of 10%

101   Is strongly predicted when fetal weight > 4 kg

With regard to the aetiology of pre-eclampsia:

102 The interstitial trophoblast has been shown to be abnormal

103 There is a decreased sensitivity to angiotensin II

104 There is a three- to fourfold increase in the risk of developing pre-eclampsia if a first-degree relative has been affected

105 Placental hypoperfusion occurs as a result of a decrease in intervillous blood flow

106 There is a raised incidence in women who change partners after the birth of their first child

In pregnancy-induced hypertension:

107 The fourth Korotkoff sound corresponds most closely with intra-arterial pressure

108 The commonly used hypertensives, labetolol, methyldopa and nifedipine, all cross the placenta

109 The use of calcium supplementation reduces the risk of pre-eclampsia

110 The use of antihypertensives has reduced the incidence of pre-eclampsia and perinatal mortality rates

111 There is good evidence for the use of low-dose aspirin to reduce the risk of pre-eclampsia

OBSTETRIC QUESTIONS

In hyperemesis gravidarum:

112   Dextrose 5% should be started until oral fluids are tolerated

113   A metabolic acidosis is characteristically seen

114   Wernicke's encephalopathy is the result of vitamin B_{12} deficiency

115   Of patients 50% have abnormal liver function tests

116   An elevated T_4 (thyroxine) and low TSH should be corrected with antithyroid medication

With regard to inflammatory bowel disease in pregnancy:

117   Active disease at the time of conception is associated with an increased risk of miscarriage

118   The risk of preterm delivery is increased if there is active disease during pregnancy

119   Azathioprine is contraindicated in pregnancy

120   Active perianal disease at the time of delivery is an indication for caesarean section

121   Pregnancy exacerbates symptoms in most cases

With regard to regional anaesthesia in labour:

122   Local anaesthetics block C-fibres at lower concentrations than Aδ-fibres

123   Opioids block C-fibres at lower concentrations than Aδ-fibres

124   Spinal doses of local anaesthetic are ten times the dose required for epidural anaesthesia

125   The incidence of dural puncture headaches is 2%

126   Epidural analgesia does not increase the need for Caesarean section

Maternal smoking in pregnancy is associated with:

127 A reduction in fetal blood flow to the brain

128 An increased risk of placental abruption

129 An increased risk of pre-eclampsia

130 A reduction in fetal breathing movements

131 An increased risk of fetal hypoglycaemia

With regard to type 1 diabetes in pregnancy:

132 It complicates 1% of pregnancies

133 Diabetic nephropathy increases the risk of fetal growth restriction and preterm delivery

134 Rapid normalisation of blood glucose levels in pregnancy is associated with an improvement in retinopathy

135 The risk of macrosomia is related to maternal postprandial glucose levels

136 Tight glycaemic control in labour improves fetal outcome

In type 1 diabetes:

137 The incidence of chromosomal abnormalities is increased

138 There is an increased rate of miscarriage

139 Anencephaly is more common

140 Serial fetal Doppler assessments are of value in assessing fetal well-being

141 Uterine artery blood flow is affected by diabetic glycaemic control

OBSTETRIC QUESTIONS

With regard to the HELLP (haemolysis/elevated liver enzymes/low platelet count) syndrome:

142   Of patients 30% occur during the second trimester

143   It can be diagnosed only in the presence of hypertension

144   Coagulation parameters are usually abnormal

145   Caesarean section may increase transaminase levels

146   It has a recurrence risk of 5%

With regard to amniocentesis:

147   Sampling failure rate is 5%

148   It is complicated by chorioamnionitis in 5% of cases

149   It may cause platelet isoimmunisation

150   It is associated with limb deformities

151   The culture failure rate is 2%

The following clinical signs in a newborn lower the Apgar score:

152   Pallor

153   Fetal pulse > 120 beats/min

154   Respiration > 30/min

155   Absence of a Moro reflex

156   Irregular respiration

In monochorionic diamniotic twin pregnancies:

157 The twins are monozygotic

158 The twins may be dizygotic

159 The presence of arterial anastomoses is protective against twin–twin transfusion

160 There is an increased incidence of cerebral palsy

161 Fetofetal transfusion syndrome complicates 5% of monochorionic pregnancies

Asymptomatic bacteriuria in pregnancy:

162 Is seen in 10% of women

163 If left untreated, will progress to symptomatic infection in > 50% of women

164 Is associated with preterm delivery

165 Is associated with low birthweight

166 Is more common in pregnancy than in non-pregnant women

Rubella in pregnancy:

167 5% of parous women are not immune

168 Is associated with IUGR

169 Is associated with congenital deafness only if infection is acquired before 16 weeks' gestation

170 Is associated with microcephaly

171 Is associated with thrombocytopenia

OBSTETRIC QUESTIONS

With regard to uteroplacental Doppler assessment:

172   It is best performed using continuous-wave Doppler

173   Normal pregnancies show a reduction in the pulsatility index

174   High-resistance velocity waveforms are seen in pregnancies at high risk of pre-eclampsia

175   High-resistance velocity waveforms are seen in pregnancies at high risk of IUGR

176   It is a good indicator of fetal hypoxia

With regard to ultrasonography in pregnancy:

177   The lambda sign distinguishes a monochorionic from a dichorionic pregnancy

178   Routine ultrasound dating will reduce induction rates

179   Routine screening has poor sensitivity for the detection of cardiac malformations

180   In spina bifida the lemon sign is more commonly seen after 24 weeks' gestation than the banana sign

In toxoplasmosis in pregnancy:

181   It is caused by a bacterium

182   Seventy per cent of infants are asymptomatic at birth

183   The severity of fetal infection is less the later it occurs in pregnancy

184   The absence of fetal IgM excludes infection

185   Maternal treatment with spiramycin reduces the risk of fetal infection

Congenital infection with CMV:

186   Affects up to 2% of live births

187   Is associated with hydrocephalus

188   Is associated with IUGR

189   Occurs only with primary maternal infection

190   May be confirmed by culture of an infant's urine

Listeriosis in pregnancy:

191   Is diagnosed by confirmation of positive serology

192   Is a water-borne infection

193   Is associated with meningoencephalitis in the neonate

194   May present as a rash at birth

195   Is associated with contamination of the amniotic fluid with meconium

Parvovirus B19:

196   Is an RNA virus

197   Results in viraemia after 1 week

198   Produces the characteristic rash during maximum viraemia

199   May cause fetal hydrops

200   May be associated with myocarditis

In Down's syndrome:

201   The chromosomal abnormality is more likely to be caused by a translocation than a non-dysfunction

202   There is an increased risk of translocation with increasing maternal age

203   If the child has a trisomy, the risk of having another affected child is 2%

204   If the child has a translocation, the risk of having another affected child is higher if the father rather than the mother carries the balanced translocation

205   If the child has a translocation, the risk of having another affected child is 10% if the mother carries the balanced translocation

Appendicitis in pregnancy:

206   The incidence is lower in pregnancy

207   The mortality rate is higher in pregnancy

208   Conservative treatment is advised if the pregnancy is less than 24 weeks

209   Maternal and fetal mortality rates are very low if perforation has not occurred

Pancreatitis in pregnancy:

210   Is more common during the third trimester

211   Presents with gallstones in over 50% of cases

212   Should be managed surgically

213   Can be diagnosed with cholangiopancreatography

214   Is associated with hyperparathyroidism

In normal pregnancy, the following coagulation factors are increased:

215 Factor X

216 Factor VII

217 Factor IIa

218 Factor XII

219 Plasma fibrinogen

Fetal hydrops:

220 Is caused by red cell isoimmunisation in most cases

221 Is the result of a chromosomal abnormality in most non-immune cases

222 Warrants recommendation of amniocentesis

223 Has a worse prognosis if there are large pleural effusions

224 Has the best prognosis if it occurs in association with fetal arrhythmias

225 Resulting from parvovirus is an indication for a termination of pregnancy

Multiple Choice
Questions: Answers

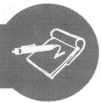
1F   2F   3T   4F   5F

Recurrent vulvovaginal candidiasis is defined as four mycologically proven episodes in 1 year. It affects a minority of cases. Other species such as *Candida glabrata* can cause it. It is difficult to treat, needing repeated antifungal treatments.

6T   7F   8T   9T   10T

The Mirena coil is not licensed for this. The COCP can be used but is no longer in use because it has been replaced by levonorgestrel.

11T   12T   13T   14F   15F

Diabetes mellitus and endometrial cancer are not complications of assisted conception.

16F   17T   18T   19T   20T

Women with one or more previous pregnancies are more at risk.

21F   22T   23T   24F   25T

A copper IUCD is the most effective emergency contraception and is not contraindicated in nulliparity. It can be fitted up to 5 days after the day of earliest predicted ovulation.

Questions on pages 3–21

26F   27F   28F   29F

The overall pregnancy rate after progesterone-only emergency contraception is 11%. It is not contraindicated in deep vein thrombosis, unlike the Yuzpe method. Established pregnancy is a contraindication and it can be used more than once in a cycle.

30T   31F   32T   33F   34T

Sexual intercourse and the use of spermicides with diaphragms are strongly associated with urinary tract infections. In children up to 1 year of age, as many as 11% of girls and 12% of boys will suffer a symptomatic urinary tract infection. It is more common in non-secretors of histoblood group antigens than in secretors.

35F   36F   37F   38T   39F

The normal parameters are a residual urine volume of < 50 ml, a first desire to void between 150 and 200 mL, and a capacity of > 400 ml. There should be no/minimal rise in detrusor pressure during filling and, if the detrusor pressure rises > 15 cmH_2O, this is diagnostic of low compliance. It is normal to have a rise in detrusor pressure on voiding of < 50 cmH_2O with a peak flow rate > 15 ml/s for a voided volume of 150 ml.

40F   41T   42F   43T   44T

Although cystoscopy is not a useful diagnostic tool, it may be used to exclude other causes of symptoms. An increase in bladder wall thickness (> 5 mm) is reported in women with detrusor overactivity. Most cases in women are idiopathic, but obstruction resulting from prostatic hypertrophy in men is a significant aetiological factor.

45T   46T   47T   48T

Risk factors for ectopic pregnancy include previous tubal pregnancy and surgery, previous PID, current IUCD users, induced abortion, assisted conception, salpingitis isthmica nodosa, smoking, diethylstilbestrol exposure, luteal phase defects and ovulatory dysfunction.

49T   50T   51F   52T

In congenital adrenal hyperplasia, the female fetus is exposed to low levels of androgen, and so partial masculinisation occurs. Complete development of male external genitalia will occur if the androgen levels are high enough.

53T   54T   55F   56T   57F

Complete moles usually contain only paternal DNA and are therefore androgenic. Most complete moles are homozygous 46XX, from the duplication of a single sperm in an ovum lacking maternal genes. Some 25% of complete moles are heterozygous, 46XY or 46XX. Partial moles are usually triploid, and an embryo may be present or inferred from the presence of fetal red cells in the villous vasculature. Partial moles can transform into choriocarcinomas.

58T   59F   60F   61F   62T

The transverse colon is most likely to be injured during laparoscopy. In cases of bladder perforation the bladder should be repaired in two layers using polyglycolic or polyglactin sutures. Non-absorbable sutures should not be used because they increase the risk of stone formation. Insertion of the Verress needle into the bladder does not require further treatment or catheterisation, provided that it is recognised and the patient is voiding well.

63F   64F   65T   66T

After stopping the combined pill, 98% of women will ovulate by their third cycle. Only 1% of women will be amenorrhoeic 6 months after stopping the combined pill.

67T   68T   69F   70F   71T

Staging of cervical cancer includes cystoscopy, proctoscopy, cervical/tumour biopsy and intravenous pyelography.

72F   73F   74T   75T   76F

Tumour size, differentiation and node involvement are important prognostic factors. Survival after surgery is closely related to tumour volume. In stage III disease the carcinoma involves the lower third of the vagina and/or extends to the pelvic side wall. Barrel-shaped tumours that expand the endocervix are associated with a higher treatment failure rate. Pelvic exenteration should be considered for central recurrences after radiotherapy.

77F   78T   79F   80F   81F

Some 70% of women have advanced disease at the time of presentation. CA-125 may be raised in both mucinous and serous tumours, as well as in other non-malignant conditions. The prognosis and treatment of ovarian cancer are related to clinical stage, amount of residual tumour and the degree of tumour differentiation. Stage IV disease is defined by the presence of malignant cells in the cytological fluid of pleural fluid, not just by the presence of a pleural effusion.

82F 83F 84T 85F 86T

Bacterial vaginosis is more common in black than in white women. The prevalence is 12–15% in UK populations. It is more common in sexually active woman, but can also be seen in virgins and lesbians. The pH is usually higher than 4.5.

87T 88F 89F 90F 91T

Neisseria gonorrhoeae is a Gram-negative diplococcus. The incubation period is short at 2–5 days. Reliable serological tests have not been developed.

92F 93T 94F 95T 96T

The risk is increased in older women and if the uterine size is greater than expected for gestational age. The risk is increased in those who have used the combined pill before evacuation because the hormones in the combined pill are probably growth factors for trophoblastic tumours.

97F 98T 99T 100F

They account for 2–4% of all ovarian tumours. Some 5–10% of cases arise in continuity with recognisable endometriosis.

101T 102F 103T 104F 105T

Some 10% of epithelial tumours are borderline, and of these the most common are mucinous (30%), followed by serous tumours. The 5-year survival rate for serous borderline tumours is 90–95%, whereas that for mucinous tumours is 81–91%.

106T   107F   108F   109F   110T

Between 5 and 10% arise from a fibroid, and these have a better prognosis than those that arise in normal myometrium. Some 20% are seen in nulliparous women. There is no increased risk in Afro–Caribbean women.

111T   112T

HIV infection rates are rising among heterosexuals. Women seem to be more vulnerable to the infection than men.

113T   114F   115T   116T   117T

Hypoplastic left heart is a major structural defect.

118T   119T   120T   121T   122F

Vaginal delivery should be the aim. Caesarean section is for obstetric reasons only.

123F   124T   125T   126F   127F

Tocolysis is contraindicated in antepartum haemorrhage because it may endanger the lives of the mother and the fetus.

128F   129T   130T

It is a Gram-positive organism.

131F   132T   133T   134T

It is common in Afro–Caribbean, Asian, Middle Eastern and Mediterranean races.

135T   136T   137F

It is not always secondary to a physical cause.

138T   139F   140T   141T

Congenital cleft lip and palate may be seen with trisomy 13 and 18 and triploidy. It is associated with the use of phenytoin and carbamazepine.

142F   143T   144F   145T   146F

Up to 70% of patients with SLE will have a flare-up of disease during pregnancy. Anti-Ro antibodies are present in 30% of patients. Cutaneous neonatal lupus develops in 5% of babies of anti-Ro antibody-positive mothers and congenital heart block in 2%.

147F   148F   149F   150F   151T

Symptoms of rheumatoid arthritis will improve in up to 75% of women during pregnancy. There is an increased risk of exacerbation of symptoms post partum. Rheumatoid arthritis does not have an adverse effect on pregnancy and there is no increased risk of miscarriage.

152T   153F   154T   155T   156T

Peripartum cardiomyopathy usually presents as heart failure late in pregnancy, the early postpartum period or up to 6 months post partum. The diagnosis is made by excluding all other causes of heart failure. It is more common in multiparous, black, relatively old and socially deprived women. In addition to antifailure treatment, these patients require anticoagulation.

157F   158F   159F   160F

During pregnancy the plasma volume starts to increase from the first trimester by 50% of its prepregnancy level by term. Most of this rise occurs by the second trimester. The heart rate and pulse volume also increase. Diastolic murmurs are uncommon and indicate functional or anatomical cardiac abnormalities.

161F   162F   163F   164F   165T

Engagement of the head occurs when the biparietal diameter passes the pelvic inlet. Active management of labour reduces the length of labour, but not the incidence of Caesarean section. Amniotomy does not affect the perinatal mortality rate or the operative delivery rate.

166T   167F   168T   169T   170T

Anti-D prophylaxis should be given after a miscarriage to all RhD-negative non-sensitised women if gestation is > 12 weeks or < 12 weeks where there has been heavy repeated bleeding or use of intrauterine instrumentation.

171F   172F   173T   174F   175F

There is a low risk of bacterial endocarditis during delivery, but most women are also given prophylactic antibiotics to reduce this risk. These patients usually have a normal cardiac reserve. There is an increased risk of teratogenicity from warfarin use, especially between 6 and 9 weeks' gestation.

176T   177F   178F   179F   180T

Up to 19% of fetuses with an abdominal circumference and estimated fetal weight less than the fifth centile have chromosomal defects. Some 50% of normally formed stillbirths are SGA. The ratios of head circumference to abdominal circumference and femur length to abdominal circumference are poorer than abdominal circumference or estimated fetal weight alone in predicting the SGA fetus or neonatal.

181F   182F   183F   184F

The incubation period is 10–21 days. Shingles in pregnancy does not result in fetal sequelae. There is no good evidence that varicella immunoglobulin prevents intrauterine infection. Fetal varicella syndrome may be detectable on ultrasonography, but congenital varicella generally occurs after 36 weeks' gestation and has no obvious ultrasonic features.

185F   186F   187T   188F   189T

The values of the amniotic fluid index at 28, 34 and 40 weeks are 90–220, 80–240 and 70–180 mm, respectively. Amniotic fluid is increased in upper gastrointestinal obstruction as a result of the inability to swallow. It is increased in neuromuscular defects caused by the neuromuscular loss of swallowing.

190T   191T   192T   193F   194F

Reduced movements and hydrops can occur with anaemia from rhesus disease; however, the absence of these features does not exclude severe anaemia. The survival rate after intrauterine transfusion is 70–75% in a hydropic fetus, but 90–95% in a non-hydropic fetus.

195T   196F   197T   198T   199T

Uterine atony is the most common cause for postpartum haemorrhage, but it can also occur as a result of a haemostatic defect or platelet deficiency. FFP should be given on the basis of clotting results. Most women tolerate a loss of 1500 ml before blood pressure drops. The aim of resuscitation should be to restore the circulating blood volume to a CVP of 5 cmH_2O.

200F   201F   202F   203T   204T   205F

Herpes gestationis is a bullous eruption in pregnancy, which clinically looks similar to herpetic lesions but is not caused by a herpes virus. Diagnosis is made by direct immunofluorescence, demonstrating C3 complement deposition at the basement membrane. Treatment is with topical corticosteroids and antihistamines. Systemic steroids are often required and should not be withheld during pregnancy.

206T   207T   208F   209F   210F

Complication rates after Caesarean section are similar in HIV-positive and HIV-negative women. Higher viral loads lead to an increased risk of vertical transmission; however, there is no threshold value at which viral transmission will not occur. The British HIV Association recommends that combination antiretroviral therapy should be started if the woman herself needs treatment (ie a viral load $> 10\,000$–$20\,000$ copies/ml and a CD4 count $< 20 \times 10^6$), as would be recommended in a non-pregnant woman. Otherwise, a twice-daily zidovudine regimen should be commenced between 28 and 32 weeks' gestation, continued until delivery and also given to the infant until 6 weeks post partum. Breast-feeding increases the risk of transmission from 15% to 30% in the UK.

211T   212F   213T   214T   215F   216T

In a monochorionic twin pregnancy, the death of one twin results in a 25% risk of cerebral damage and a 25% risk of death in the surviving twin.

217F   218T   219T   220T   221F

The standard deviation is the square root of the variance. The mean may be higher or lower than the mode, depending on which way the data are skewed.

222T   223F   224F   225T

The following table should be constructed to calculate sensitivity, specificity and negative and positive predictive values:

PRACTICE PAPER ANSWERS

	With the condition (bladder cancer)	Without the condition
Screen positive	True positive (a)	False positive (b)
Screen negative	False negative (c)	True negative (d)

1.   The sensitivity of the test is the probability that the test is positive if the condition is present = $a/(a + c)$ (= 50%).

2.   Specificity is the probability that the test will be negative if the condition is absent = $d/(b + d)$.

3.   The negative predictive value is the probability that the condition is absent if the test is negative = $d/(c + d)$.

4.   The positive predictive value is the probability that the condition is present if the test is positive = $a/(a + b)$.

ANSWERS TO GYNAECOLOGY PRACTICE QUESTIONS

1F 2T 3F 4F 5T

The incidence of mild, moderate and severe dyskaryosis is 5, 1 and 0.5%, respectively. The cervical screening programme targets women aged between 25 and 64 years.

6T 7T 8T 9T 10F

The aetiology of anal sphincter injury is multifactorial and vaginal delivery is a significant aetiological factor. Episiotomy, particularly midline episiotomy, is a significant risk factor, as well as fetal macrosomia, the use of forceps over a Ventouse, an occipitoposterior position and a prolonged second stage. Elective Caesarean section has been shown to reduce the risk of anal sphincter injury, but there is evidence that occult anal sphincter injury can occur after Caesarean section during the second stage.

11T 12F 13T 14F

Faecal incontinence is more common in women than in men, and the incidence increases with age. Anal sphincter injury after vaginal delivery is the most significant aetiological factor. Pudendal neuropathy recovers in most women after vaginal delivery and is not related to symptoms.

GYNAECOLOGY ANSWERS

Questions on pages 23–39

15F   16F   17T   18F

There is no evidence that faecal incontinence after delivery is reduced by elective episiotomy. Risk factors for the development of symptoms after a history of a previous third-degree tear include vaginal delivery in a symptomatic woman, presence of a sphincter defect of more than one quadrant, and an increment of < 20 mmHg in anal squeeze pressures.

19F   20F   21F   22F

Conservative therapy should always be considered in the first-line management of stress incontinence. However, the success of pelvic floor exercises is variable – reported at between 27 and 90% – and dependent on patient compliance and motivation. Most studies have not reported long-term success rates. Alpha-Agonists have moderate effects but are not routinely used, and their use is limited by side effects. Oestrogen therapy has not been shown to be of use in women with stress incontinence. Electrical stimulation acts by stimulating the pudendal nerve, leading to contraction of the pelvic floor.

23F   24T   25F   26T   27F

An anterior repair should not be considered for the treatment of stress incontinence. The tension-free vaginal tape procedure has a similar 5-year success rate as Burch colposuspension. Burch colposuspension, but not the Marshall–Marchetti–Krantz procedure, will correct a coexistent cystocele. Needle suspension procedures have a low long-term success rate of approximately 18%.

28F   29F   30T   31F

Premature ovarian failure occurs in 1% of women under 40 years of age. Most of the cases are idiopathic, but it is also related to chromosomal disorders (eg Turner's syndrome, gonadal dysgenesis), metabolic defects (galactosaemia, 17 alpha-hydroxylase deficiency), immunological disorders (DiGeorge's syndrome) and autoimmune disorders (pelvic tuberculosis and mumps oophoritis). Pelvic surgery and chemotherapy or radiotherapy will also lead to premature ovarian failure. Primary amenorrhoea is seen in 25% of cases, and occurs in 15% of patients with secondary amenorrhoea.

32T   33F   34F   35F   36F

One-third of cases of azoospermia are the result of non-obstructive causes, and these cases should have karyotyping performed. The other cases are caused by obstruction, and in these cases a testicular biopsy usually shows normal spermatogenesis. Azoospermia is reported in 15% of infertile men.

37F   38T   39F   40F

The frequency of malignant tumours is 13% in premenopausal women and 45% in postmenopausal women. Mature cystic teratomas are the most common tumours leading to torsion, occurring in 3.5–10% of cases. Some 2% of ovarian torsions involve ovarian malignancy.

41T   42T   43T   44T

Rupture occurs most commonly on days 20–26 of the ovarian cycle. Haemorrhage into a cyst is more common on the right than the left side, possibly as a result of cushioning of the left ovary by the rectosigmoid colon, or the increased intraluminal pressure on the right side from the differential ovarian vein anatomy. Excessive bleeding may cause haemolytic jaundice.

45F   46T   47T   48T   49F

The risk of ovarian hyperstimulation syndrome is related to young age, low body weight, polycystic ovaries, high dose of gonadotrophins, large number of retrieved oocytes, high estradiol level on the day of hCG administration, use of luteal support and ensuing pregnancy.

50T   51T   52F   53F

The ectopic pregnancy rate varies between 2 and 11%, and a heterotopic pregnancy is estimated to occur in 1% of IVF pregnancies.

54F   55T   56T   57F

The ovulation rate in a normally oestrogenised woman is reported at between 60 and 85%. The use of clomifene citrate is associated with a 50% increase in endogenous FSH and LH.

58F   59T   60F   61F

GnRH analogues are synthesised by substitution of amino acids at positions 6 and 10 of the decapeptide GnRH. After an initial increase in gonadotrophin and oestrogen levels, most women will be hypo-oestrogenic within 2–3 weeks of starting treatment.

62T   63F   64F   65T

In the situation of 21-hydroxylase deficiency, the precursor 17-hydroxyprogesterone accumulates and diverts precursors to androgen synthesis, leading to increased levels of urinary pregnanetriol, ketosteroids and serum testosterone. Aldosterone synthesis is defective.

66F   67T   68T   69F

Endocrine changes associated with the menopause include a decrease in oestrone, oestradiol and androstenedione. Gonadotrophin, cholesterol and calcium levels increase, but there is no change in plasma testosterone.

70T   71F   72T   73F   74T

Turner's syndrome is the most common sex chromosome abnormality. Its phenotype is related to the loss of sex chromosome material – short stature, coarctation of the aorta, broad chest, widely spaced nipples and renal anomalies such as horseshoe kidney. As a result of ovarian dysgenesis, the gonadotrophin levels are raised and oestrogen levels are decreased. There does not seem to be a relationship to increased maternal age.

75F   76T   77T   78T   79F

Secondary causes of hyperprolactinaemia include hypothyroidism and drugs that interfere with dopamine synthesis, release or reuptake. It is also seen in association with renal failure and acromegaly. Around 20% of patients will have non-functioning pituitary adenomas, which increase prolactin levels by stalk compression rather than by an increase in secretion.

80F   81F   82T   83F   84T

Well-controlled diabetes mellitus and treated thyroid disease are not associated with recurrent miscarriage. Balanced or reciprocal translocations are the most frequently detected parental chromosomal abnormality. Robertsonian translocations are less frequent, occurring in 1% of couples with recurrent miscarriage.

85T   86T   87T   88F   89T

Precocious puberty is defined as the onset of puberty before the age of 8 years in girls and before the age of 9 years in boys. Causes of precocious puberty include: idiopathic (family history and overweight/obese); intracranial lesions, gonadotrophin-secreting tumours, congenital brain defects (neurofibromatosis, third ventricle cysts), hypothyroidism; and gonadotrophin-independent conditions, such as congenital adrenal hyperplasia, Cushing's disease, McCune–Albright syndrome, sex steroid-secreting tumours (adrenal or ovarian), chorion epithelioma and exogenous oestrogen ingestion/administration.

90F   91F   92F   93T   94T

Total serum testosterone levels are raised in only 40% of women, and levels do not correlate well with the severity of hirsutism or acne. The DHEAS level reflects adrenal androgen secretion and is normal in over 50% of cases.

95T   96T   97F   98F   99T

The half-life is approximately 19 hours. The failure rate is dependent on age, being almost as low as that for the combined pill in those aged over 35 years. The failure rate is higher in those who weigh > 70 kg; therefore such women should be advised to take two pills a day.

100T   101F   102T   103T   104F

Hyperthyroidism and hypogonadism are associated with osteoporosis.

105T   106T   107F   108T   109T

Pathological hyperprolactinaemia may be caused by drugs that inhibit dopamine action or production, eg phenothiazines, butyrophenones, methyldopa, cimetidine and pimozide.

110T   111F   112T   113F   114F

Gonadotrophin levels are lower in Kallmann's syndrome, anorexia nervosa and McCune–Albright syndrome.

115T   116F   117F   118F   119F

There is much experimental evidence for the aetiological role of certain high-risk human papillomaviruses – HPV-16, -18, -31, -33, -35, -45, -51, -52, -58 and -59. The HPVs are non-enveloped DNA viruses. Regions E6 and E7 code for oncoproteins, which interfere with cell-cycle regulation.

120F   121T   122T   123T   124F

Risk factors include early age at first intercourse, multiparity, multiple sexual partners, other genital tract neoplasia, previous CIN, combined oral contraceptive and certain dietary factors.

125F   126F   127T

Cervical intraepithelial neoplasia may affect the gland crypts and the epithelium. The mean depth of crypt involvement is 1.25 mm.

128T   129F   130F   131T   132T

Only 50% of patients show a glandular abnormality on cytology. In two-thirds of patients there is an invasive squamous lesion or CIN.

133F   134F   135T

Forty per cent of women are aged under 40 years. Between 20 and 45% of patients are asymptomatic.

136T   137F   138T   139T

In patients with atypical hyperplasia, a coexistent carcinoma is found in 25–50% of cases. Cystic hyperplasia is a common finding, with a risk of progression to endometrial carcinoma of 0.4–1.1%.

140T   141F   142T   143F   144F

The risk of progression of vulvar intraepithelial neoplasia (VIN) is 5–10%. Paget's disease is associated with concomitant genital tract malignancy in 20% of cases. The risk of malignant transformation of lichen sclerosus is 3–5%.

145T   146T   147F   148F   149F

Stage I lateralised lesions may be managed with a wide local excision. In superficial lesions the groin nodes do not need to be removed, because they are rarely involved. Elderly women have a higher incidence of nodal disease.

150T   151T   152T   153T

Malformations associated with diethylstilbestrol exposure include a classic T-shaped uterus with widening of the isthmic and interstitial portions of the fallopian tube and narrowing of the lower third of the uterus, as well as non-specific uterine abnormalities with changes in the cavity.

154F   155F   156T   157F   158T

Krukenberg's tumours occur as secondaries from primary tumours in the gastrointestinal tract, eg stomach, colon, gallbladder or bile duct. They often secrete oestrogen but not progesterone or gastrin.

159T   160F   161T   162T

A knowledge of toxicity of commonly used chemotherapy is essential. Cisplatin can cause ototoxicity, nephrotoxicity and peripheral neuropathy. Neurotoxicity is a common side effect with vincristine. Doxorubicin can cause cardiomyopathy, leading to heart failure and this risk is dose related.

163T   164F   165F   166T   167T

Germ-cell tumours include dysgerminomas, endodermal sinus tumours (yolk sac), embryonal cell tumours, polyembryoma choriocarcinomas, teratomas and mixed tumours. Brenner's tumour and endometrial tumours are of epithelial origin.

168T   169T   170F   171T

Serous cystadenocarcinoma is the most common ovarian tumour. Psammoma bodies are noted in 30% of cases. Bilateral involvement is seen in 30–50% of cases.

172F   173T   174T   175F   176T

5 alpha-Reductase deficiency occurs as a result of a mutation in the short arm of chromosome 2. Virilisation occurs at puberty. Production of testosterone and anti-Müllerian hormone from the testes is normal. Affected individuals have ambiguous genitalia and are born with predominantly female or ambiguous genitalia (often clitorophallus, bifid scrotum and vagina).

GYNAECOLOGY ANSWERS

177F   178T   179F   180F

Old age, obesity, abdominal distension, chest infection, malignancy and jaundice increase the risk of wound dehiscence. The mass closure technique, but not tension sutures, reduces risk. A non-absorbable suture should be used because catgut loses its tensile strength over 10 days and polyglycolic acid loses most of its strength within 21 days.

181T   182F   183F   184F   185T

The ureter is made up of three layers and lined with transitional epithelium. It is retroperitoneal in the abdomen, passes along the anteromedial aspect of psoas major and is crossed by ovarian vessels. It enters the pelvis anterior to the sacroiliac joints and crosses the bifurcation of the common iliac artery, and passes along the posterolateral aspect of the pelvis running in front of and below the internal iliac artery. It then travels in the base of the broad ligament and is crossed superiorly and medially by the uterine artery, entering the bladder at the trigone.

186F   187F   188F   189F   190T

The bladder has a rich parasympathetic supply and this is derived from cell bodies in the grey columns of S2–S4. There is little sympathetic innervation of the bladder. Parasympathetic action is mediated via acetylcholine acting on muscarinic receptors. Sympathetic nerves originate from T10–L2 and mediate their action via α-receptors and β-receptors.

191F   192T   193F   194T   195T

Non-closure of the peritoneum at caesarean section is recommended because it is associated with lower postoperative febrile morbidity and less use of postoperative analgesia. Peritoneal closure increases the risk of bladder adhesions after Caesarean section. Peritoneal closure after vaginal hysterectomy is not recommended because there is no evidence from trials to date of any benefit.

196T   197F   198F   199T

The risk of malignancy in these cysts is less than 1%. Some 50% will resolve within 3 months. It may be reasonable to manage these cysts conservatively, depending on the patient's symptoms.

200T   201F   202F   203T   204F

Some 85% of viable intrauterine pregnancies show a 66% rise in beta-hCG every 48 hours in the first 40 days of gestation, but only 13% of all ectopic pregnancies show this rise. A beta-hCG rise of < 50% in 48 hours is strongly associated with a non-viable pregnancy, irrespective of the site of gestation. The value of serum progesterone measurement is equivocal, because there is overlap between normal and ectopic pregnancies. A level > 25 ng/ml is associated with a normal intrauterine pregnancy in 98% of cases.

205F   206T   207F   208F   209F

The peak incidence is between 30 and 45 years. It is more common in monozygotic than in dizygotic twins. Dysmenorrhoea is the most common presenting symptom affecting 60–80% and dyspareunia is reported in 25–40%.

210T   211T   212T   213T   214T

Danazol has side effects related to its androgenic and anabolic properties, including weight gain, acne, oily skin, hot flushes, depression and mood changes. Skin rashes, hirsutism and deepening of the voice, leucopenia and thrombocytopenia, and cholestatic jaundice are also seen, albeit less commonly.

215T   216F   217T   218F   219T

Gestrinone has a high affinity for progesterone receptors and also binds to androgen receptors, but not to oestrogen receptors. It abolishes the mid-cycle gonadotrophin surge but has no significant effect on basal levels. Some 85–90% of patients are amenorrhoeic within 2 months.

220F   221T   222T   223F   224F   225F

The main aetiological factors for endometrial cancer are obesity, unopposed oestrogen and hormone replacement. Nulliparity increases the risk two- to threefold, and late age at menopause also increases the risk. Smoking and the combined pill decrease it. Progestogens protect the endometrium.

ANSWERS TO OBSTETRIC PRACTICE QUESTIONS

1F   2F   3F   4T

A positive family history is found in up to 50% of patients, and family studies suggest an autosomal dominant mode of inheritance. The risk of stillbirth does not correlate with the level of serum transaminases, but it may be related to the maternal serum concentration of bile acids. Doppler studies are not useful in predicting fetal risk.

5F   6F   7T   8T   9T

Pathological adherence of the placenta – as in placenta accreta, increta or percreta – is associated with previous surgical procedures to the uterus, including Caesarean section and uterine curettage.

10F   11F   12F   13F   14T

Fetal alcohol syndrome is associated with the characteristic facies of microcephaly, growth retardation, renal and cardiac abnormalities, and mental handicap.

15F   16T   17F   18T

ITP is an autoimmune disease causing purpura during pregnancy. It is confirmed by the presence of an increased number of megakaryocytes in the bone marrow. Bleeding problems are unlikely unless the platelet count falls to < 50 000/mm³.

Questions on pages 41–57

19F   20T   21T   22T   23T

The umbilical vein carries oxygenated blood from the placenta to the fetus. It then flows through the liver to the ductus venosus and the inferior vena cava. Blood passes through the foramen ovale into the left atrium before it is ejected from the left ventricle into the ascending aorta. Deoxygenated blood returns to the placenta via the umbilical artery.

24T   25F   26F   27T   28F

A raised serum maternal AFP level may be found in women with exophthalmos, gastroschisis and Turner's syndrome. It may also be raised after fetomaternal transfusion, eg after a threatened abortion or amniocentesis. It is reduced in Down's syndrome pregnancies.

29T   30F   31F   32F   33T

Routine scanning for second trimester anomalies in the UK detects 25% of cases with congenital defects and 30–50% with trisomy 21. It almost never detects cerebral palsy.

34T   35F   36T   37T   38F

Neonatal jaundice in the first 24 hours after birth is a result of blood group incompatibility. Jaundice is associated with galactosaemia where there is a deficiency of galactose-1-phosphate uridyltransferase. Phenylketonuria is not associated with jaundice. Sickle cell disease may cause jaundice in the older child but not in the neonate. Neonatal jaundice is also seen in association with hypothyroidism.

39F   40F   41F   42T   43T

CMV is the most common cause of congenital infection in the UK, and is more common in lower socioeconomic groups. Infection can occur via perinatal transmission or sexual transmission or from blood products. Transplacental passage can occur in both primary and secondary infections. The highest risk of transmission is when infection occurs during the first trimester. Only 5–10% of babies infected with CMV at birth are symptomatic.

44F   45F   46T   47T   48T

Face presentation occurs in 1 in 1500 births. It results in the presentation of the submentobregmatic diameter at the pelvic brim – the diameter of which is similar to the suboccipitofrontal diameter of a flexed vertex. The mentoanterior position is more favourable for vaginal birth. Face presentation is associated with anencephaly, pelvic malformation and prematurity.

49F   50F   51T   52F   53F

The plasma volume increases by 50% in pregnancy and the red cell mass by 18%. Ferrous sulphate causes more gastrointestinal side effects than ferrous gluconate. There is no evidence that routine iron supplementation improves the pregnancy outcome for women on a healthy diet, but it may do so for those in developing countries where there is a higher level of maternal anaemia. There is no effect on the risk of postpartum haemorrhage, pre-eclampsia and antepartum haemorrhage.

54F   55T   56F   57T   58F

Congenital adrenal hyperplasia has an autosomal recessive mode of inheritance. Marfan's syndrome and familial hypercholesterolaemia have an autosomal dominant pattern of inheritance.

OBSTETRIC ANSWERS

59F   60T   61F   62T

A loud, third heart sound will be detected on auscultation, not on an ECG. The P–R interval is not changed.

63F   64T   65F   66F   67T

The cerebellum is abnormal in 70% of cases. Some 95% of babies with neural tube defects have abnormalities of the head, such as hydrocephalus, abnormal head shape (lemon shape) and abnormal cerebellar shape (banana shape). The maternal serum acetylcholinesterase level is normal in a closed spina bifida, but raised in an open neural tube defect. Antenatal limb movement is not a good predictor of limb function postnatally.

68T   69F   70T   71F   72F

Fetal breathing movements are increased by maternal caffeine and glucose intake. At 26 weeks' gestation, the normal fetus spends 8% of its time breathing when it is active and 2% when quiet; at 34 weeks' gestation, this is 34% and 26%, respectively, and at 40 weeks' 28% and 16%, respectively. A biophysical profile is less accurate in predicting fetal compromise in cases of maternal diabetes than pregnancies complicated by other pathologies because the increase in amniotic fluid seen in diabetes overrides the other markers. Fetal breathing movements usually decrease 72 hours before the onset of labour as a result of fetal arterial prostaglandin E levels.

73T   74F   75F   76T

The umbilical artery waveform indices are dimensionless. They are independent of the angle of insonation. The resistance index depends on the maximum frequency shift during diastole (A), in diastole (B) and is calculated as $(A - B)/A$. The resistance index is 1 when there is reversed or absent flow.

77F   78T   79F   80T   81F

Hyperthyroidism occurs in 0.2% of pregnancies and hypothyroidism in 2.5%. Thyroid peroxidase antibodies are associated with hyperthyroidism. There is a 50% chance of postpartum thyroid dysfunction if a woman has thyroid peroxidase antibodies in early pregnancy.

82T   83F   84F   85T   86F

There is no indication for measurement of cervical length in a woman with a previous first trimester miscarriage or after a previous LLETZ (large loop excision of the transformation zone) or cone biopsy.

87T   88T   89F   90F   91F

Maternal sex steroids predominate in the fetal circulation. The fetus synthesises its own insulin and controls its own thyroid and adrenal function.

92F   93F   94T   95F   96F

Vesicovaginal fistulas are more common than rectovaginal ones. They usually present between day 3 and day 10, after the devitalised area has sloughed off. Fistulas should not be repaired immediately because some will close spontaneously. They should be managed conservatively for up to 8 weeks to allow spontaneous closure, and also to let any infection and oedema settle, which, of course, increase the chance of successful healing of any surgical procedure. The route of surgery depends on the surgical access achievable: a suprapubic route should be used when vaginal access is difficult. The success of fistula repair is related to good surgical technique and healing.

OBSTETRIC ANSWERS

97F   98F   99T   100F   101F

Shoulder dystocia occurs in 1 in 300 deliveries. It occurs when the bisacromial diameter is greater than the pelvic inlet. The risk of recurrence is < 5%. As only 20% of shoulder dystocia cases occur in babies weighing > 4 kg, estimated fetal weight is therefore not a strong predictor.

102F   103F   104T   105T   106T

In pre-eclampsia, the endovascular trophoblast invasion is defective whereas the interstitial trophoblast invasion is normal. There is an increased sensitivity to angiotensin II. It is thought that there is a decrease in fetal tolerance to paternally derived antigens. Avoidance of barrier methods of contraception and a longer period with the same partner reduce the risk, because this may increase exposure to paternal antigens in the sperm.

107F   108T   109T   110F   111F

The Korotkoff sound V corresponds best with intra-arterial pressure and is the most reproducible end-point in pregnancy. Calcium supplementation at a dose of 2 g/day has been shown to reduce the risk of pre-eclampsia, but it has no effect on perinatal mortality rates. Large randomised trials have shown little or no therapeutic benefit of low-dose aspirin. However, a subanalysis of the CLASP (Collaborative Low-dose Aspirin) trial showed that low-dose aspirin taken before 16 weeks' gestation reduces the incidence of early onset pre-eclampsia in high-risk women.

112F   113F   114F   115T   116F

Physiological or 0.9% saline is the fluid of choice because 5% dextrose can result in hyponatraemia. A metabolic alkalosis is characteristically seen. As hCG is a weak thyrotrophin agonist it may result in a rise in T_4 and a lowering of TSH early in pregnancy. These levels normalise as pregnancy progresses and hCG levels decrease. Unless there are clinical signs of hyperthyroidism, the patient does not need treatment.

117T   118T   119F   120T   121F

Azathioprine, steroids and 5-aminosalicylic acid are safe to use during pregnancy. If the disease is well controlled, pregnancy does not worsen it. However, 60% of patients will continue to have symptoms if active disease is present at the time of conception.

122F   123T   124F   125F   126T

Local anaesthetics block conduction in Aδ-fibres at concentrations lower than those needed to block C-fibres. The reverse is seen with opioids. Epidural doses of local anaesthetic are 10 times higher than those required for spinal anaesthesia. Dural puncture occurs in < 1% of patients, 70% of whom will develop a severe low-pressure headache as a result of cerebrospinal fluid leakage.

127F   128T   129F   130T   131F

Smoking is related to a decreased risk of pre-eclampsia. It also causes a decrease in fetal breathing movements but not blood flow to the brain. Smoking increases the risk of placental abruption and placenta praevia. The risk of miscarriage, preterm labour and IUGR is related to smoking in a dose-dependent fashion. It is not associated with fetal hypoglycaemia.

132F   133T   134F   135T   136T

Type 1 diabetes complicates 1 in 300 pregnancies. Rapid normalisation of the blood glucose level in pregnancy causes a transient progression in retinopathy. The pre-pregnancy control, speed of control and extent of pre-existing retinopathy are related to the risk of progression. There is a close relationship between intrapartum glucose control and fetal hypoglycaemia.

OBSTETRIC ANSWERS

137F   138T   139T   140F   141F

The risk of congenital, but not chromosomal, abnormalities is increased. Uterine artery blood flow is not affected by glycaemic control, nephropathy or vasculopathy. Fetal Doppler measurements are of limited value because in these pregnancies there is not the redistribution of flow seen in cases of IUGR.

142F   143F   144F   145T   146F

Some 15% of cases occur during the second trimester. The HELLP syndrome (haemolysis, elevated liver enzymes, low platelets) complicates 20% of cases of severe pre-eclampsia. In 15% of cases with the HELLP syndrome there is no hypertension or proteinuria. The coagulation parameters of prothrombin time, partial thromboplastin time and serum fibrinogen time are usually normal. Mode of delivery has been shown to affect transaminase levels, with levels rising more after Caesarean section than after vaginal delivery. The recurrence rate is 19–27%.

147F   148F   149F   150F   151F

The sampling failure rate is < 2% and the culture failure rate is as low as 0.3%. Chorioamnionitis complicates up to 1% of cases and is a cause of miscarriage. Amniocentesis is not associated with limb deformities.

152T   153F   154F   155F   156T

A fetal heart rate of 120/min and a respiratory rate of 30/min each have an Apgar score of 2. Pallor scores 0. Irregular respirations score 1. Reflex activity is tested by grimace on stimulation, not by the Moro reflex.

157T   158F   159T   160T   161F

Monochorionic twins are monozygous not dizygous. There is a 10–15% risk of fetofetal transfusion, and hence an increase in the risk of fetal brain lesions and cerebral palsy.

162F   163F   164T   165T   166F

Asymptomatic bacteriuria is seen in 3–8% of pregnant women. It is not more common in pregnancy but it is more likely to progress to symptomatic infection. If left untreated, there is a 25% chance of symptomatic infection and pyelonephritis. As there is an association with preterm delivery and low birthweight, it is standard practice to screen women routinely at each antenatal visit.

167F   168T   169F   170T   171T

Some 12% of parous women are non-immune. Congenital deafness is noted even with late infection up to 20 weeks' gestation.

172F   173T   174T   175T   176F

Continuous wave Doppler is a blind investigation, whereas colour Doppler allows identification of the uterine artery and is therefore more accurate and reproducible. With increasing gestational age there is a reduction in resistance to blood flow within the uterine arteries. This is seen as a fall in the resistance and pulsatility indexes of the Doppler waveform, and the early diastolic notch also disappears. The high-resistance waveform persists in pregnancies in which there is defective trophoblastic invasion, such as pre-eclampsia and IUGR.

177F   178T   179T   180F

At 6–9 weeks' gestation there is a thick septum between the two sacs of a dichorionic pregnancy, which thins but is still identifiable as a thick septum at the base of the membrane – the so-called 'lambda sign'. Dating by menstrual dates is inaccurate in 70% of cases, so dating by ultrasonography would reduce the number of inductions performed for 'post-term' pregnancies. In spina bifida, the lemon sign is a result of deformity of the frontal bone and is reliably seen up to 24 weeks' gestation. The banana sign, caused by abnormal cerebellar shape, is seen in almost all cases from 15 weeks' gestation onwards.

181F   182T   183T   184F   185T

Toxoplasmosis is caused by the protozoan *Toxoplasma gondii* and is usually asymptomatic. Some 70% of infected infants are asymptomatic but may later develop chorioretinitis, blindness, strabismus, hydrocephaly, microcephaly, cerebral calcification, deafness, and mental handicap and psychomotor retardation. These infants should be followed up for at least 2 years. The risk of fetal infection is lower in the first trimester. However, if it does occur it results in more severe disease. Fetal IgM is not produced till after 19 weeks' gestation and therefore early fetal blood samples may be unreliable.

186T   187T   188T   189F   190T

CMV infection is the most common cause of intrauterine infection. Although it is more common after primary maternal infection, it can also occur after recurrent infection. Congenital infection can lead to growth retardation, hepatosplenomegaly, chorioretinitis, haemolytic anaemia and intracranial calcifications.

191F   192F   193T   194T   195T

Listeriosis is diagnosed from cultures of blood and other sources, such as genital tract swabs and urine. It can arise from the ingestion of contaminated food such as soft cheese and pâté.

196F   197T   198F   199T   200T

Parvovirus B19 is a DNA virus. Transmission is via respiratory and nasal secretions. The rash typically appears 17–18 days after infection and after the virus is no longer present.

201F   202F   203T   204F   205T

Most cases are the result of trisomy from non-dysfunction caused by meiotic errors during ovum formation. About 5% of cases are the result of translocation where there are 46 chromosomes, but one of these chromosomes is abnormal. This abnormal chromosome arises from the centric fusion of one chromosome with another acrocentric chromosome, such that the resultant child is trisomic for chromosome 21 and has two independent chromosomes, the third being fused to another chromosome. Increased maternal age increases the risk of non-dysfunction. If the father carries the balanced translocation, the risk of recurrence is lower than if the mother carries it.

206F   207T   208F   209T

The incidence is similar in pregnant and non-pregnant women. The mortality rate is 17% if perforation has occurred and is higher than in non-pregnant women. The diagnosis is often difficult to make and so treatment is often delayed. Surgery should be performed when clinically indicated, even if the fetus is not viable.

210T   211T   212F   213F   214T

Most cases of pancreatitis resolve with conservative management, and this should be the first option. Cholangiopancreatography should not be performed in pregnancy because of the high radiation risk.

215T   216T   217F   218F   219T

Normal pregnancy is accompanied by increases in the levels of factors VII, VIII and X, as well as fibrinogen.

220F   221T   222T   223T   224T   225F

The incidence of non-immune hydrops is 1 in 1000 and the ratio of non-immune to immune hydrops is 9:1. The diagnosis is based on a generalised skin oedema, and collections of fluid in at least one visceral cavity. If there is only one fluid-filled serous cavity, a thick placenta should also be seen for diagnosis. If it is caused by parvovirus it can resolve spontaneously.

Essay Writing Tips

The examination

There will be two papers of 1 hour 45 minutes and four questions each. Each question will carry equal marks. There will therefore be approximately 26 minutes to answer each question. It is important that you do not spend too much time on one question at the expense of another.

An analysis of past papers between 1997 and 2002 (10 papers) indicates that two-thirds of the questions involve management of clinical problems or a clinical scenario, eg:

> A 26-year-old woman in her first pregnancy requests a detailed scan at 18 weeks' gestation and the baby is found to have a single choroid plexus cyst. Discuss the implication of this finding and justify your management.

The other third of questions are more factual, eg:

> Discuss routine pregnancy dating.

The common instructions are 'justify' (20%), 'counsel/advise' (20%), 'describe/summarise' (16%), 'evaluate' (12%) and 'critically analyse' (12%).

You must take into the examination two black pens – ballpoints are preferable to fountain pens – a ruler and an accurate watch.

Preparation

This book is not intended to teach you obstetrics and gynaecology but to assist you in the technique required to express your knowledge in the format necessary to pass the examination. Hard work is the key to achieving the standard required and there are no short cuts.

The examination itself will rely on the standard management applicable to British obstetric and gynaecological practice. It will not test research knowledge or knowledge of new or untried techniques or developments. You would, however, need to be up to date with new developments, provided that they have found a place in current clinical practice.

Most of your preparation will come from standard texts in obstetrics and gynaecology, and up-to-date reviews found in journals: *The Obstetrician and Gynaecologist* (publication of the Royal College of Obstetrics and Gynaecology or RCOG), *Current Obstetrics and Gynaecology* and *The Green Top Guidelines* published by the RCOG.

In addition to an appropriate level of knowledge in the subject, it is necessary to practise some questions so that flaws in technique can be improved and the ability to write concisely with acceptable handwriting perfected.

Over the years we have seen numbers of extremely good doctors with an excellent knowledge of the subject fail the examination repeatedly because of the inability to conform to the timing, structure and format that the examination demands.

Practice questions

Technique

It is essential that you write in sentences; notes or lists are not acceptable. If there are a number of facts that need to be given they can be given as a sentence using commas, eg:

> The symptoms of endometriosis include lower abdominal pain, dyspareunia, dysmenorrhoea and infertility.

It is essential to underline the headings necessary to give the examiner an idea of the structure that you have applied to your answer. *Do not* underline words in the text.

Underline the word at the start of the sentence, eg the above sentence should be written:

> Endometriosis is associated with symptoms of lower abdominal pain, dyspareunia, dysmenorrhoea and infertility.

It is essential to use a ruler to underline and do not underline too many words because the emphasis will be lost.

Writing

It is essential to write legibly. The examiner will not waste time reading a scribbled answer.

What you consider to be good writing may not be easy for others to read and it is advisable that you give your practice answers to someone else to check.

If your writing is of a borderline standard, it is advisable to write your headings in block capitals so key words will stand out. Thus the above sentence could be written:

ENDOMETRIOSIS is associated with symptoms of lower abdominal pain, dyspareunia, dysmenorrhoea and infertility.

Remember, with respect to handwriting, that quality not quantity is important.

Timing

There are 26 minutes allocated to each question and you must not go over time. If your answer is well structured and planned, you will have been awarded most of the marks before the end of the question is reached. If the answer is well structured, you have begun your answer with the most important aspects and received most of the marks. The last part of your answer may not gain many marks because it is a less important aspect of the topic being discussed. It makes no sense to compromise the next answer by going over time writing down minutiae on an answer. The examiners will not see all of your answers together, so you will not be given any sympathy for running short of time and failing to complete an answer.

Read the question

The anxiety, adrenaline and tension of the moment have led many candidates to misread the question. This is a common problem and may result in failure of an otherwise acceptable paper. You must read, and then re-read, the question before making your answer plan, and then again after making it.

Answer plan

It is essential that you do a rough answer plan before you start your answer. The plan should take only a few minutes to complete and, together with re-reading the question, should ensure that you do not make a large omission or unusual interpretation of the question. Many candidates do not wish to 'waste time' on an answer plan, but this is a false economy, because not only does it allow you to formulate your answer but it also enables you to structure the answer so that you start with the most important details. You also get an idea of the scope of your answer and how much detail you need in order to finish in 26 minutes.

Structuring your answer

It is important to structure your answer; this can be achieved by using your answer plan. Once you have a structure, enter the details of your answer in each section of the plan.

Break down your answer

It is important, as part of your answer plan, that the question is broken down into constituent parts to enable you to structure your answer. The following are examples:

First trimester–second trimester–third trimester (in 'outline the antenatal care of a woman with cardiac disease in pregnancy').

First stage–second stage–third stage (in 'outline the intrapartum care of a woman with cardiac disease in pregnancy').

History–examination–special investigations (in 'discuss the differential diagnosis of a woman with deep dyspareunia').

Preoperative–intraoperative–postoperative (in 'discuss the ways of reducing the incidence of wound sepsis associated with an abdominal hysterectomy').

Stage 1–stage 2–stage 3–stage 4 (in 'outline the management of ovarian cancer').

Immediate–delayed–long term (in 'describe the complications of radiotherapy when used to treat cervical cancer').

Medical–laparoscopic–open surgical (in 'evaluate the treatment of severe endometriosis').

It is necessary to plan, break down and structure each question.

Motto

Quality not quantity

'Do's

1.   Read and then re-read the question.

2.   Write a brief answer plan.

3.   Structure your answer.

4.   Underline key headings at the start of a paragraph.

5.   Write in sentences.

6.   **Finish EACH question on time.**

'Don't's

1.   Write in note form.

2.   Give long lists without explanation.

3.   Underline in the text of your answer.

4.   Go overtime on any question.

5.   Scribble.

Essay questions

1. A 34-year-old, nulliparous woman has been found to have a pelvic mass. Ultrasonography confirmed the presence of multiple uterine fibroids. Critically appraise your management.

2. A 42-year-old, multiparous woman presents with a 6-month history of intermenstrual bleeding (IMB). Justify your investigations.

3. A 25-year-old, obese woman has noticed excessive hair growth over the past 12 months. Discuss your further management.

4. Critically appraise the different options available for the surgical treatment of menorrhagia.

5. Urinary incontinence represents a major health problem for many women. Justify your diagnostic steps.

6. Surgical treatment of vulval carcinoma may cause significant postoperative morbidity. Describe measures that can be taken to avoid this.

7. Outline the benefits of the levonorgestrel intrauterine system (Mirena coil).

8. Compare and contrast the treatment options for symptomatic endometriosis.

9. Review the effects of medical treatment for the relief of menopausal symptoms.

10. Laparoscopically assisted vaginal hysterectomy should be the preferred method for removal of the uterus. Debate this statement.

11. Ovarian hyperstimulation syndrome (OHSS) is a potentially severe complication of supraphysiological ovarian stimulation. Outline the measures that can be taken to prevent OHSS.

12. You are called to theatre by your Senior House Officer (SHO) who was about to perform a termination of pregnancy (TOP) at 12 weeks' gestation, but reports that he has perforated the uterus. You are the most senior doctor available. How would you deal with this situation?

13. Discuss the impact of diagnostic radiology on the management of gynaecological patients.

14. Outline the investigation and treatment of a couple with recurrent miscarriages.

15. A patient is admitted with hyperemesis gravidarum at 10 weeks' gestation. Describe your management plan.

16. Discuss the epidemiology of gynaecological cancers and how to reduce their incidence.

17. A 23-year-old, primigravid woman has a scan at 30 weeks' gestation, which shows severe intrauterine growth restriction (IUGR). Discuss your further management.

18. Discuss the impact of prepregnancy clinics on future obstetric outcomes.

19. Describe the management of a patient with chronic renal failure at 10 weeks' gestation.

20. A 32-year-old woman attends the antenatal clinic. She is known to be HIV positive. She is now 14 weeks' pregnant and wishes to discuss the implications of HIV in pregnancy. How would you counsel her?

21. A 26-year-old primigravida is admitted at 27 weeks' gestation, semi-conscious and with a history of convulsions. Outline the possible causes and principles of management.

22. A 45-year-old, grand-multiparous woman presents at 7 weeks' gestation in the antenatal booking clinic. Formulate a management plan specific to her pregnancy.

23. A multiparous woman remains in the second stage of labour for 2 hours despite having good uterine contractions. At pelvic examination the fetal head is found to be in the occipitotransverse position. Justify your decision on the mode of delivery.

24. Compare and contrast the different drugs available for thromboprophylaxis in pregnancy.

25. Describe the complications of Caesarean section and discuss the possible methods of prevention.

26. A 29-year-old, primigravid woman presents at 28 weeks' gestation with marked oligohydramnios. Justify your investigations.

27. A woman has had a failed trial of rotational forceps delivery and is now prepared to be delivered by emergency Caesarean section. Give a detailed account of the measures that you would implement to ensure a safe delivery.

28. A 33-year-old woman has had two second trimester losses in the past. She is now 13 weeks' pregnant and requests cervical cerclage. Would you support her request?

29. Describe the management of a patient with acute fatty liver at 32 weeks' gestation.

30. A patient is 32 weeks' pregnant and has obstetric cholestasis. Describe your approach to her management.

31. Discuss the causes and management of disseminated intravascular coagulation (DIC) in obstetrics.

32. A 30-year-old woman arrives at a routine antenatal visit at 20 weeks' gestation smelling of alcohol. She admits to drinking excessively throughout her pregnancy. Discuss your further management.

Essay answers

Gynaecology

Essay 1
A 34-year-old, nulliparous woman has been found to have a pelvic mass. Ultrasonography confirmed the presence of multiple uterine fibroids. Critically appraise your management.

Essay tips
The key words in this question are:

- 34 year old, nulliparous – fertility

- pelvic mass – the nature of the mass (multiple uterine fibroids), confirmed by ultrasonography – so not a diagnostic question.

Essay plan
Critically appraise management:

- history of symptoms (menstrual/pressure/dyspareunia/quality of life), fertility

- examination, size, etc.

- special investigations: ultrasonography, computed tomography, (CT), magnetic resonance imaging (MRI), haemoglobin (Hb) urea and electrolytes (U&Es)

- treatment: conservative, total abdominal hysterectomy (TAH), myomectomy (hysteroscope/laparoscope), medical (hormonal/ non-hormonal).

Specimen essay (340 words)

History of the problems caused by the fibroids, eg quantity of menstrual loss, subfertility, pelvic pain, urinary and/or bowel symptoms, as well as their impact on her life, should be taken into account.

Examination for the signs of anaemia should be sought, followed by an abdominal examination to assess the size and mobility of the fibroid mass.

A speculum vaginal examination to inspect the cervix and a bimanual pelvic examination are needed to confirm the size and mobility of the uterus.

Investigations should include a full blood count (FBC) as well as iron studies if there is anaemia. An intravenous urogram, CT or MRI may rarely be needed if other organs are compressed or diagnosis is unclear.

Treatment depends on the presenting signs and symptoms, and the wishes and expectations of the patient.

Conservative management is possible in a completely asymptomatic patient.

Tranexamic acid and/or mefenamic acid may be considered for a woman with small fibroids and menorrhagia.

Gonadotrophin-releasing hormone (GnRH) analogues improve haemoglobin levels. A 3-month course may shrink fibroids by as much as 40–60%, which might make future myomectomy easier. However, these drugs are expensive, cause menopausal symptoms and can be used for only a short time.

The oral contraceptive pill is cost-effective, may reduce menstrual loss and is useful if the patient wants contraception.

Myomectomy may be considered if subfertility is a problem and the fibroids are the only identifiable cause, either by hysteroscopy for submucous fibroids or by laparoscopy for subserous and pedunculated fibroids.

Open myomectomy carries a small risk of hysterectomy and postoperative adhesions. Good haemostasis and intraoperative vasopressin may help to prevent this.

Subtotal or total hysterectomy is the definitive treatment for fibroids. However, it may not be acceptable to this particular woman if fertility is desired.

Uterine artery embolisation is another option open to this woman. The procedure is effective in over 60% of cases. There is a 1–2% risk of loss of ovarian function. At present it is not considered suitable for women intending to embark on a future pregnancy.

Essay 2

A 42-year-old, multiparous woman presents with a 6-month history of intermenstrual bleeding (IMB). Justify your investigations.

Essay tips

The key words in this question are:

- 42 years of age

- multiparous

- 6 months

- justify (why would you do that and what is the evidence)

- investigations (not treatment and not management).

Essay plan

- History:

    – detailed menstrual history (postcoital bleeding), obstetric history, more children?

    – sexual, social, contraception, drugs, treatment, hormones, menopause, family history of cancer.

- Examination: thyroid, diabetes, pelvic pathology.

- Investigations: ultrasonography (abdominal/vaginal), hysteroscopy, D&C (dilatation and curettage), Doppler, colposcopy.

Specimen essay (293 words)

Intermenstrual bleeding describes bleeding between periods.

Menstrual history should include details of: the bleeding, how heavy it is, and when it occurs in relation to her cycle; drug use (eg tamoxifen), contraception (eg Depo-Provera).

Past gynaecological, medical and surgical history should be enquired about to elicit problems, eg diabetes, thyroid disease, uterine/cervical/ovarian surgery, menopausal symptoms.

General examination including signs of anaemia, or goitre, tachycardia, exophthalmos could point towards thyroid dysfunction.

Gynaecological examination is needed to look for cervical and uterine pathology, eg cervical lesions, inflammation, adnexal masses.

Investigations include an FBC and thyroid function tests if the history suggests.

A cervical smear should be taken and a high vaginal and endocervical swab for *Chlamydia* and other sexually transmitted pathogens.

Transvaginal ultrasonography (TVS) including saline diffusion sonography (to improve diagnostic accuracy and detect endometrial polyps) may help diagnose fibroids.

An endometrial Pipelle biopsy should be obtained to exclude endometrial hyperplasia or malignancy.

Colposcopy should be performed and a directed biopsy taken if the cervix appears suspicious or the patient has a history of abnormal smears. If carcinoma of the cervix is diagnosed, the patient should undergo an examination under anaesthesia (EUA) and staging.

Doppler studies of the ovarian vessels and endometrium may be considered if there are any suspicious sonographic features in these organs.

Hysteroscopy and directed biopsy is the investigation of choice over the traditional D&C because the latter is blind, samples less than 50% of the cavity and can miss polyps.

If adnexal masses are found then further investigations, such as pelvic ultrasonography and Doppler scans, CA-125 and diagnostic laparoscopy may be necessary.

Extragenital sources of bleeding: if the bleeding is found to originate from the bowel or the renal tract then a mid-stream urine sample (MSU), cystoscopy or a sigmoidoscopy should be arranged.

Essay 3

A 25-year-old, obese woman has noticed excessive hair growth over the past 12 months. Discuss your further management.

Essay tips

The key words in this question are:

- 25 years of age – obese

- excessive hair growth

- 12 months

- discuss

- management.

Essay plan

- History: menses, virilisation, drugs, galactorrhoea, contraception, infertility, family history of malignancy, racial.

- Examination: body mass index (BMI), visual fields, virilisation, hair pattern.

- Investigation: androgen profile, thyroid-stimulating hormone (TSH), prolactin (PRL), pelvic ultrasonography, screen for Cushing's syndrome.

- Treatment: oral contraceptive (OC), Dianette, cyproterone, dexamethasone, spironolactone cosmetic treatments.

Specimen essay (309 words)

Hirsutism is most commonly caused by benign aetiological conditions. However, malignant tumours of the ovaries and adrenal glands or Cushing's syndrome should not be overlooked. Polycystic ovarian disease (PCOD) appears to be the likely cause in this case.

History of menstrual cycles, the presence of headaches, visual field disturbances and galactorrhoea. The racial background and a family history of hirsutism should be defined.

A drug history is also important, eg danazol.

Gynaecological examination should be performed, paying particular attention to signs of virilism, eg temporal balding, deepening of the voice, breast atrophy and clitoromegaly or, alternatively, a Ferriman–Galway score.

Cushingoid features, eg buffalo neck, should be sought.

Pelvic examination should focus on adnexal masses, although androgen-secreting ovarian tumours may be too small to palpate.

Pelvic ultrasonography should detect adnexal masses.

Hormonal profile taken, including: early to mid-follicular phase luteinising hormone (LH), follicle-stimulating hormone (FSH), PRL, testosterone, dehydroepiandrosterone sulphate (DHEAS), 17-hydroxyprogesterone, thyroid function and sex hormone-binding globulin (SHBG). A serum testosterone level > 6 nmol/L should prompt a search for an ovarian tumour or adrenal hyperplasia, therefore necessitating use of CT or MRI.

A 24-hour urinary free cortisol estimation and blood pressure if Cushing's syndrome is suspected.

Treatments should include the following:

Weight loss increases SHBG levels and reduces bioavailable testosterone.

The oral contraceptive pill will treat mild hirsutism, especially Dianette, which contains the anti-androgen cyproterone acetate (CPA). This increases SHBG levels and regulates the menstrual cycle.

Sequential regimen of CPA 50–100 mg may be useful for the more severe cases. Pregnancy should be avoided for 3 months after the cessation of treatment.

Spironolactone may be useful; patients should have electrolyte levels, especially potassium, monitored regularly.

Dexamethasone 0.5 mg will help to control raised DHEAS levels.

Tumours of the ovaries or adrenals should be treated surgically.

Cosmetic treatment such as waxing, peeling, shaving and electrolysis may be offered.

Essay 4

Critically appraise the different options available for the surgical treatment of menorrhagia.

Essay tips

The key words in this question are:

- critically appraise (pros and cons of each method)

- different options

- available (not experimental)

- surgical treatment (not medical)

- menorrhagia.

Essay plan

Different options:

- total abdominal hysterectomy/subtotal hysterectomy

- laparoscopically assisted vaginal hysterectomy (LAVH)

- vaginal hysterectomy

- D&C

- endometrial ablation – diathermy, microwave, thermal, laser.

Specimen essay (323 words)

Patient selection is vitally important because haemorrhage, infection and thromboembolism may complicate surgical procedures. These complications need to be balanced against the treatment of a benign condition.

Hysterectomy is the definitive treatment of menorrhagia.

Laparoscopically assisted vaginal hysterectomy enables a total abdominal hysterectomy (TAH) to be transformed into a vaginal hysterectomy (VH), or a difficult VH into an easy one. Although the operating time is prolonged, it compares favourably with VH in terms of patient recovery, time, reduced pain relief and shorter hospital stay. It is the method of choice in associated suspected adnexal mass and endometriosis, and adhesiolysis can be performed.

Vaginal hysterectomy gives an improved cosmetic result. Oophorectomy can be successfully performed in 95% of patients. Severe post-operative morbidity is higher than with TAH as shown in the VALUE (Valsartan antihypertensive long-term use evaluation) study.

Total abdominal hysterectomy or a subtotal hysterectomy, has the advantage of easy access and good vision of structures such as uterus and bladder/bowel; if needed, it affords easy oophorectomy. The patients, however, may incur other intraoperative or postoperative morbidity, including cosmetic effects of a scar. Costs caused by prolonged hospital stays and prolonged pain relief are relevant. There is a risk of haemorrhage, thromboembolism and infections.

Endometrial ablation/resection can be performed in a number of ways, eg by diathermy, or microwave, thermal or laser techniques.

Endometrial resection is useful for women who have completed their family and can be performed as a day-case procedure. However, patient satisfaction and amenorrhoea rate are less than with TAH, and dysmenorrhoea cannot be cured. The risk is intraoperative fluid retention, causing pulmonary oedema, coma and death. Haemorrhage, infection and pregnancy complications can occur, and endometrial cancer might be easily overlooked in the future.

Endometrial ablation is easier and does not have the problems related to fluid overload, may be performed under local anaesthesia, is quicker to learn and produces similar results.

D&C is not recommended because it provides no more than temporary relief from menorrhagia.

Essay 5
Urinary incontinence represents a major health problem for many women. Justify your diagnostic steps.

Essay tips
The key words are:

- urinary incontinence

- a major health problem for many women

- justify

- diagnostic steps (no marks for therapy, and note *not* diagnostic tests).

Essay plan

- History: symptom complex, severity, health impact.

- Examination – prolapse, demonstration of incontinence.

- Investigations:

  – volume voiding chart, pad test, MSU

  – cystoscopy, videocystourethrography, cystometry

  – pressure profile, flow studies, electromyogram (EMG).

Specimen essay (316 words)

Appropriate investigations in urogynaecology are largely determined by the information elicited from the history and the examination findings.

History of incontinence, the duration of the symptoms, frequency, urgency and nocturia, as well as haematuria, need to be established. The patient's age, occupation, presence of chest conditions, constipation, drug history (eg diuretics), and drinking and smoking habits should be recorded.

The effect on her social life should be assessed, and sexual activity and associated gynaecological problems noted.

A gynaecological examination should focus on the mobility of the anterior vaginal wall and the presence of pelvic masses and demonstration of incontinence.

Speculum examination may reveal genital atrophy, a pool of urine might be visible in the case of a fistula and a coexistent cystocele or rectocele can be detected with a Sims speculum examination.

An MSU for culture and sensitivity testing should be taken from a patient with classic frequency, urgency and dysuria.

A pad test can provide a quantitative assessment of the amount of urinary loss in women with mild symptoms

A fluid/volume chart is cheap, simple and informative, may clarify the patient's drinking habits, eg tea, coffee, and should form a baseline investigation.

Cystoscopy and an intravenous urogram to rule out malignancy and other serious pathology, eg interstitial cystitis.

Urodynamics is the standard investigation. Detrusor overactivity might be better detected by ambulatory urodynamics and additional tests such as ultrasonography for bladder wall thickness.

Urethral pressure profilometry may detect urethral instability, whereas a dual channel cystometry can generally differentiate stress from urge incontinence types.

Video-cystourethrography is particularly helpful in patients with previous failed surgery or vesicoureteric reflux.

Flow studies might be performed before planned surgery because a low flow rate increases retention problems after surgery.

An electromyogram should be done for patients with suspected neuropathy and/or myopathy. CT or MRI is useful in further characterising pelvic masses.

Urethrocystography can be performed if a fistula is suspected.

Essay 6

Surgical treatment of vulval carcinoma may cause significant postoperative morbidity. Describe measures that can be taken to avoid this.

Essay tips

The key words in this question are:

- surgical treatment

- vulval carcinoma

- postoperative morbidity

- describe measures.

Essay plan

- Preoperative: counselling, treatment of medical diseases.

- Input from anaesthetists/psychologists?

- Intraoperative: appropriate incisions, haemostasis with wound drains, antibiotics and thromboprophylaxis.

- Postoperative: regular reviews, mobilisation, early recognition of complications, communication with nurses, physiotherapists and dietitians.

Specimen essay (317 words)

Referral within 2 weeks to a cancer centre not only allows input from an expert multidisciplinary team, but also reduces significant disease progression.

Preoperatively: oncology counselling nurse input and good communication with the patient and the primary health team may help to reduce psychological morbidity.

Medical and drug history should be obtained, and physician and anaesthetist involvement considered if there are coexisting medical problems. Any coexisting gynaecological disease, eg a prolapse, should be assessed.

Basic investigations and full preoperative work-up should include an FBC, blood for group and save, U&Es and a chest radiograph. An intravenous urogram and ECG may also be required.

Intraoperative: sterile surgical technique and an in-depth anatomical knowledge are important.

Thromboprophylaxis as well as meticulous haemostasis and drains will facilitate the patient's recovery.

Antibiotic prophylaxis is indicated.

Early stage vulval cancer may be managed with a wide local excision and unilateral groin node dissection; no groin dissection is necessary in stage Ia.

Simple vulvectomy with bilateral groin node dissection over separate incisions is, however, needed in patients with central vulval cancer, and achieves similar results to radical vulvectomy and lymphadenectomy. The former procedure is, however, associated with much less postoperative wound complications, anatomical distortion and lymphoedema. Therefore, a wide local excision instead of a V (butterfly) incision is preferable.

If superficial groin lymph nodes are found to be positive on frozen section histology, the deep groin nodes should also be removed.

Postoperative: early mobilisation and physiotherapy may help to prevent thromboembolism, decubitus ulcers and pneumonia.

Limb elevation and massage, in addition to prolonged suction drainage, may help to reduce the risk of lymphoedema secondary to groin dissection.

Antibiotic therapy and nursing care may help to prevent wound breakdown/infection.

Reviews of management will permit early detection of complications.

Psychological support and sexual counselling may reduce morbidity caused by changed body image.

Regular follow-ups are important so that early treatment can be instituted for recurrences.

Essay 7

Outline the benefits of the levonorgestrel intrauterine system (Mirena coil).

Essay tips

The key words in this question are:

- outline (tests factual knowledge)

- benefits (not the side effects/complications)

- Mirena coil.

Essay plan

- contraception: high risk/over age 40

- fertility

- menstrual loss: fibroids, endometriosis

- endometrial hyperplasia

- PMS (premenstrual syndrome)

- PID (pelvic inflammatory disease).

Specimen essay (219 words)

The Mirena coil is a relatively newly developed IUCD impregnated with the progestogen levonorgestrel.

Effective contraception is a major advantage (Pearl index).

Fertility quickly returns to normal once it has been removed.

Contraception in high-risk women where oestrogen is contraindicated, eg in thromboembolic, cardiac or diabetic patients, is a major advantage over many other methods.

Contraception in the over-40 age group is a major use, especially in patients with coexisting menorrhagia.

Improving menstrual disorders: Mirena has gained wide acceptance for the treatment of menorrhagia and dysmenorrhoea may also improve. There are reports of significant reductions in the number of hysterectomies for benign indications, thereby leading to cost savings.

Endometrial hyperplasia is treated by the slow-release levonorgestrel, which acts locally at the endometrium. This local delivery avoids the progestogenic side effects associated with systemic administration during combined hormone replacement therapy (HRT), and in other circumstances where endometrial protection from oestrogen administration is indicated.

PMS and associated symptoms are improved by the Mirena coil, probably because of the improvement in menorrhagia and dysmenorrhoea.

Endometriosis is improved symptomatically by the reduction in menstrual flow.

PID has been found to be less common in women with a Mirena coil.

Other benefits include the prevention and treatment of fibroid-associated menorrhagia and the prevention of ectopic pregnancies.

Essay 8

Compare and contrast the treatment options for symptomatic endometriosis.

Essay tips

The key words in this question are:

- compare/contrast (give the similarities and differences of each treatment and the place in management, eg reserved for severe disease)

- treatment options

- symptomatic (include dysmenorrhoea, deep dyspareunia, pelvic pain and subfertility)

- endometriosis.

Essay plan

- Medical:

  – hormonal: oral contraceptive (OC), progesterone, danazol/gestrinone, mifepristone

  – non-hormonal: mefenamic acid, GnRH analogues.

- Surgical:

  – open – TAH/BSO (bilateral salpingo-oophorectomy)

  – minimally invasive.

- Alternative.

Specimen essay (341 words)

Treatment options may be medical, surgical or alternative, and are generally considered in the context of the patient's history, findings on physical/pelvic examination and other investigations.

Non-hormonal treatments include the prostaglandin synthetase inhibitors (eg mefenamic acid). These are effective in relieving dysmenorrhoea and pelvic pain, and have the advantage that fertility is not impaired.

Hormonal treatments are effective in providing symptom relief but they all interfere with fertility. Moreover, there is a significant chance of recurrence of endometriosis once treatment is discontinued.

The OC pill relieves dysmenorrhoea and dyspareunia and may be a suitable option for young women with mild symptoms who do not wish to become pregnant.

Progestogens achieve symptom relief in 80% of cases, but there is some concern about increasing the risk for cardiovascular disease in the long term.

Danazol given in amenorrhoeic doses improves symptoms, but is not well tolerated because of its androgenic side effects. Gestrinone given orally twice weekly is as effective as danazol, but has a better side-effect profile.

GnRH analogues are particularly effective in women with superficial lesions and relieve symptoms in 90% of women. However, it is expensive, the injection is uncomfortable, it is ineffective against endometriomas large than 3 cm and may be associated with marked vasomotor symptoms and bone loss.

Mifepristone (RU486), and tamoxifen need further clinical evaluation.

Surgery aims to restore pelvic anatomy in fertile women or to interrupt the sensory pathways in symptomatic patients; it may be performed laparoscopically or as an open procedure.

TAH and BSO may be offered to women who have completed their families and/or have coexistent gynaecological disease such as large fibroids and menorrhagia. All surgical options carry the potential risk of bleeding, infection and venous thromboembolism, and damage to the bowel, ureter and bladder.

Laparoscopic laser vaporisation or coagulation of endometriotic deposits improves fertility, whereas nerve ablation of the uterosacral ligaments achieves a 60% improvement in symptoms.

Acupuncture or hypnotherapy may work in motivated women and no side effects are known. However, their effectiveness has yet to be proved in randomised trials.

Essay 9
Review the effects of medical treatment for the relief of menopausal symptoms.

Essay tips

The key words in this question are:

- review (summarise the facts)

- effects (potential benefits and harmful effects)

- medical treatment (not surgical)

- menopausal symptoms (not menopausal problems).

Essay plan

- oestrogen

- progestogens

- tibolone

- phyto-oestrogens

- clonidine

- testosterone

- antidepressants (SERMs or selective oestrogen receptor modulators).

Specimen essay (343 words)

Over 80% of women experience at least one menopausal symptom. Medical treatment aims to prevent and/or treat these symptoms and improve quality of life with minimal adverse effects.

Oestrogens are proven to relieve vasomotor symptoms and improve urogenital symptoms and depressed moods. There is also some evidence that oestrogens might prevent, or slow, the onset of Alzheimer's disease. Randomised controlled trials (RCTs) have shown that treatment improves quality of life and well-being.

However, oestrogen therapy is associated with the short-term side effects of weight gain and breast tenderness. Long-term adverse effects include an increased risk of venous thromboembolism, endometrial cancer and breast cancer.

Progestogens have been shown to reduce vasomotor symptoms in RTCs; however, they exert no beneficial effects on bone density. Progestogens are associated with various side effects, including breast tenderness, bloating, water retention and mood changes.

Tibolone significantly improves vasomotor symptoms, libido and vaginal lubrication. Sexual satisfaction is reported to be better with tibolone than with sequential HRT. Bone density increases, but the reports of effects on psychological symptoms and quality of life are conflicting. Breakthrough bleeding occurs in about 10% of users.

Phyto-oestrogens, which may be found in soya flour, relieve the frequency and severity of vasomotor symptoms. Their effects on urogenital atrophy, psychological well-being and quality of life await further research. There are no known harmful effects.

Clonidine reduces vasomotor symptoms and has no more unwanted effects than placebo.

Testosterone improves sexual enjoyment and libido. Although reduced doses of oestrogen may be needed to control vasomotor symptoms, its effects on psychological symptoms and quality of life are undergoing further studies. There is no increase in the incidence of adverse androgenic effects when testosterone is used in approved replacement doses of 50–100 mg every 6 months.

Antidepressants and their effects on menopausal symptoms have not been thoroughly studied. However, there are well-documented harmful side effects associated with this class of drugs, including: sedation and agitation, urinary and visual problems, liver dysfunction and cardiac dysrhythmias.

SERMs can be used to maintain bone density but do not help with vasomotor symptoms.

Essay 10

Laparoscopically assisted vaginal hysterectomy (LAVH) should be the preferred method for removal of the uterus. Debate this statement.

Essay tips

The key words in this question are:

- LAVH

- should be the preferred method

- removal of the uterus (ie hysterectomy)

- debate (give the pros and cons).

Essay plan

LAVH:

- cost of equipment/duration of procedure

- blood loss/analgesia requirements

- recovery time/return to normal/cosmetic results

- surgical training

- patient selection, eg obesity, previous abdominal surgery, associated problems.

Specimen essay (301 words)

LAVH aims to convert a TAH into a vaginal procedure, or to complete a difficult VH instead of converting it into an abdominal one. By definition, the uterine vessels are divided laparoscopically.

Advantages of LAVH include good cosmetic results, reduced postoperative analgesia requirements, shorter hospital stay and a quicker return of patients to their normal activities. With respect to these, it competes favourably with VH and, despite the prolonged operation time and cost of equipment, it is still cost-effective. The average blood loss is also less than with TAH

Training of surgeons and acquisition of the necessary skills take longer for a LAVH than for TAH or VH.

Associated gynaecological problems (eg endometriosis) may be treated with an LAVH and would be the preferred method over VH, because both diagnosis and treatment can be offered at the same operation. Nevertheless, TAH is still the operation of choice for patients with large tumours, because it offers good access, visualisation and tactile information about the whole pelvis and the abdomen, as well as the opportunity for omentectomy, lymphadenectomy and easier adnexectomy.

Obese patients with previous abdominal surgery and adhesions are more at risk of complications at laparoscopy (eg damage to blood vessels and bowel), and therefore need careful assessment.

Difficulties with VH arise when there is poor access, an enlarged immobile uterus and/or suspected adnexal pathology; however, laparoscopic removal of an adnexal mass and adhesiolysis may convert a difficult hysterectomy into an easy procedure.

Laparoscopy is the 'gold standard' investigation of adnexal/pelvic pathology and has replaced laparotomy and TAH for this indication. It combines the ability of diagnosis with treatment, eg for endometriosis.

In summary, LAVH may be of benefit for some patients who would otherwise have had a TAH, but LAVH has little to add in cases where a VH is possible.

Essay 11

Ovarian hyperstimulation syndrome (OHSS) is a potentially severe complication of supraphysiological ovarian stimulation. Outline the measures that can be taken to prevent OHSS.

Essay tips

The key words in this question are:

- outline

- measures

- to prevent OHSS (not to treat)

- all of the first sentence.

The candidate is not asked to discuss or debate this statement.

Essay plan

Increased risk of OHSS?

- Young, slim, polycystic ovaries, previous history of OHSS.

To prevent OHSS:

- Non-pharmacological

    – diet, laparoscopic ovarian drill for obese women with polycystic ovary syndrome (PCOS)

    – ultrasonography, estradiol monitoring, ? cycle cancellation

    – cryopreservation of all embryos.

- Pharmacological:

    – replacement of GnRH, hMG (human menopausal gonadotrophin) regimen with FSH

    – discontinue cycle/withholding of the ovulatory hCG injection

    – use of LH instead of hCG for final follicular maturation

    – progesterone for luteal phase support

    – intravenous albumin

    – immunomodulation in the future.

Specimen essay (293 words)

Selection of patients for the prevention of OHSS starts with the recognition of their risk factors. Special attention should be paid to young and thin women, women with polycystic ovaries and women with a previous history of OHSS because these groups are at increased risk.

Referral to an expert in assisted conception in a dedicated in vitro fertilisation (IVF) unit would be the first step.

Non-pharmacological preventive measures include: a diet programme for obese patients with PCOS and laparoscopic ovarian drill for women with clomifene-resistant PCOS.

Clomifene use as first choice for ovulation induction has less risk of hyperstimulation compared with gonadotrophins.

Ultrasonography may be used to monitor ovarian response, and cancellation should be considered for cycles with excessive ovarian response (more than 12 follicles).

Measurement of serum oestradiol levels is also important in high-risk women as well as cryopreservation of all embryos that may reduce the number of hyperstimulation cycles.

Cautious use of gonadotrophins and manipulation of treatment within the pharmacological group may help to reduce severe OHSS. Purified FSH given by the low-dose incremental regimen can replace the GnRH analogue/hMG regimen. In cycles with excessive ovarian response ovulatory hCG can be withheld. Also, in cycles with high serum oestradiol levels, discontinuation of gonadotrophin administration and delayed hCG injection is effective in reducing the risk of OHSS. Recombinant LH instead of hCG should be used for final follicular maturation.

Progesterone has been shown to be as effective as hCG for luteal phase support and could be a safer option. Albumin can be given intravenously at the time of oocyte retrieval to enhance oncotic pressure and reduce the risk of OHSS.

Immunomodulation studies are currently in progress and this approach may be used in the future to prevent severe OHSS in high-risk patients.

Essay 12

You are called to theatre by your SHO who was about to perform a termination of pregnancy (TOP) at 12 weeks' gestation but reports that he has perforated the uterus. You are the most senior doctor available. How would you deal with this situation?

Essay tips

The key words in this question are:

- the scenario as described in the first two sentences

- how you would deal with this situation.

Essay plan

- History:

  - gestation

  - ? bicornuate uterus

  - blood loss

  - perforating instrument.

- Examination: size of the uterus.

- Investigation: diagnostic laparoscopy.

- Treatment: complete evacuation of uterus:

  - small hole, not actively bleeding → expectant management with oxytocics

  - moderately sized tear, moderate blood loss → laparotomy and sutures, inspection of bladder and bowel

  - large tear with massive bleeding → laparotomy, homoeostatic suture, ? proceed to hysterectomy,

  - ? involvement of bowel surgeon

- Follow-up.

Specimen essay (336 words)

A perforated, pregnant uterus represents an emergency situation.

Emergency action resuscitation starts with the placement of another intravenous line and appropriate fluid replacement. If the patient is not intubated, the anaesthetist should consider this and the patient be ventilated artificially. The appropriate arrangements for a laparoscopy and laparotomy are made.

A quick history will clarify the gestational age of the pregnancy, whether to expect a bicornuate uterus, how much blood has been lost so far and what instrument perforated the uterus.

A speculum examination will give some information about the blood loss and a bimanual examination should be performed to assess the size of the uterus.

An FBC and crossmatch of two units should be performed.

A diagnostic laparoscopy should be done swiftly to assess the size and location of the perforation and to achieve haemostasis. At the same time assurance is needed that neighbouring structures such as the bladder and bowel are intact.

Evacuation of the uterus should be completed.

A small perforation not actively bleeding may be managed expectantly, covering the patient with antibiotics and giving her oxytocics. An average-sized tear in the uterus, bleeding moderately, may be controlled by pressure. Failing that a laparotomy is required. Haemostatic sutures can be applied, and the bladder and bowel inspected for possible damage. If in any doubt, a general surgeon should be called to help.

A large perforation, bleeding massively, may necessitate a hysterectomy for haemostatic purposes, and to ensure the patient's survival. This decision should not be postponed unnecessarily but taken by senior members of the multidisciplinary team. Arrangements may need to be made to transfer the patient postoperatively to a high-dependency unit and thromboprophylaxis should be prescribed.

The risk manager, the consultant and the patient's GP should be informed as soon as possible. A clear explanation should be given to the patient and good and legible operative notes kept.

Follow-up arrangements should be made regardless of the severity of the perforation to ensure that the patient has recovered fully and also to discuss contraception.

Essay 13

Discuss the impact of diagnostic radiology on the management of gynaecological patients.

Essay tips

The key words in this question are:

- discuss

- diagnostic radiology (not radiotherapy)

- management

- gynaecological patients.

Essay plan

- pros and cons

- ultrasonography

- radiograph

- computed tomography (CT)

- magnetic resonance imaging (MRI)

- radionuclide imaging

- oncology, gynaecological endocrinology, infertility and urogynaecology.

Specimen essay (339 words)

Rapid progress has been made in the field of diagnostic radiology over the past few decades, and this field is now a cornerstone of gynaecological practice.

Ultrasound scan, either abdominal or transvaginal, assists in the diagnosis of early pregnancy, polycystic ovarian syndrome and ovarian cysts (for which Doppler might be added). Fibroids can be visualised and endometrial thickness measured in women with postmenopausal bleeding. It generally assists in the diagnosis of uterine and adnexal pathology.

Doppler ultrasonography has more recently been endorsed in the diagnosis of deep vein thrombosis.

A venogram is still the 'gold standard', despite being painful, exposing the patient to radiation and having the risk of transport of thrombus to the lungs.

A ventilation–perfusion scan is performed to diagnose or exclude pulmonary embolism – one of the main complications of gynaecological surgery.

Chest radiographs assist in the diagnosis of metastatic gynaecological disease, and also of postoperative pneumonia, pulmonary oedema and embolism. A plain film of the abdomen is used to localise a coil and to diagnose ileus postoperatively. A barium meal might be necessary in the diagnosis of chronic pelvic pain. An intravenous urogram is used in the assessment and staging of gynaecological tumours, eg hydronephrosis in cervical cancer, and also in patients with urinary incontinence.

Hysterosalpingography is used in the diagnosis of lesions associated with infertility and may help to detect a tubal patency in failed sterilisation.

Radiological investigations are well established but have the disadvantage of radiation exposure, and are potentially carcinogenic.

CT and MRI are mainly used in diagnosis and treatment planning, as well as in the detection of recurrent disease in gynaecological oncology.

The advantage of MRI is that it involves no radiation exposure at all; however, it is expensive and not universally available. Caution has to be exercised in patients with epilepsy, those who have copper IUCDs and those with myocardial infarction.

Radionuclide imaging can be used for detecting metastatic disease in bones, and also for measuring bone density. There is, however, some concern about whether these investigations might be carcinogenic.

Essay 14

Outline the investigation and treatment of a couple with recurrent miscarriages.

Essay tips

- Definition of recurrent miscarriages.

- Outline investigation and treatment.

- Investigations: ultrasonography, fetal and parental karyotypes, lupus anticoagulant or anticardiolipin antibodies.

- Those not routinely done are thyroid function tests (TFTs) and tests for diabetes.

- Treatment: aspirin, heparin and genetic counselling.

Essay plan

- Investigations:

  – karyotype ×2

  – karyotype products of conception

  – ultrasonography

  – thrombophilia

  [– endocrine not done]

  [– infective not done].

- Treatments:

  – aspirin/heparin

  – reassurance

  – genetic counselling.

Specimen essay (277 words)

Recurrent miscarriages are defined as three consecutive first trimester miscarriages. It is a distressing problem that affects 1% of all women.

Investigations

Peripheral blood karyotyping of both partners should always be performed. A balanced translocation could be present in 3–5% of couples.

Cytogenetic analysis of fetal products is useful if available or if the next pregnancy fails.

A pelvic ultrasound scan should be done to assess uterine anatomy and morphology.

A lupus anticoagulant or anticardiolipin antibody screen will reveal antiphospholipid syndrome if there are two positive test results done at least 6 weeks apart.

Tests are not routine for infective causes, thyroid or diabetes mellitus because there is no evidence of these conditions causing recurrent miscarriages.

Treatment

Genetic counselling for couples with genetic abnormalities should be arranged. A balanced translocation is the most common finding and the prognosis depends on the chromosomes involved.

Low-dose aspirin and heparin significantly improve the future live birth rate in women with recurrent miscarriages and antiphospholipid syndrome. Aspirin should be started once a positive pregnancy test has been confirmed and heparin once a fetal heart has been seen on a 7-week ultrasound scan.

Aspirin is safe in pregnancy. Heparin does not cross the placenta but may cause maternal thrombocytopenia and osteoporosis. Serial platelet counts should be done. Treatments can be stopped at 34 weeks.

Myomectomy may be offered to women with submucous fibroids and uteroplasty to those with a severe anatomical abnormality.

Reassurance should be given to couples with unexplained recurrent miscarriages who have an excellent prognosis without any treatment (75% success rate in the next pregnancy).

New or experimental treatments should be given only as part of a clinical trial.

Essay 15

A patient is admitted with hyperemesis gravidarum at 10 weeks' gestation. Describe your management plan.

Essay tips

- Definition of hyperemesis gravidarum.

- Describe: give a factual account of this common gynaecological problem.

- Management plan means history, examination, investigations and treatment.

Essay plan

- History: severity, duration, thyroid symptoms.

- Examination: dehydration, size of uterus.

- Investigations: FBC, U/E's, LFTs, ultrasonography of uterus and adnexae, TFTs, urine microscopy, culture and sensitivity.

- Treatment

  - fluids

  - antiemetics

  - steroids

  - antithyroid drugs

  - termination of pregnancy (TOP).

Specimen essay (294 words)

Hyperemesis gravidarum is defined as persistent vomiting with the patient unable to tolerate any oral food and fluids. There is a risk of dehydration, fluid and electrolyte imbalance and malnutrition. It occurs in about 1% of pregnancies and is a diagnosis of exclusion. In severe cases there may be low-birthweight babies.

History

The duration of symptoms, and what she is able to tolerate orally, are important. In addition to vomiting there may be ptyalism and spitting. Check for urinary symptoms.

Examination

Dehydration, tachycardia and postural hypotension should be noted.

Investigations

An FBC and renal, liver and thyroid function tests can reveal a raised haematocrit, deranged U&Es, abnormal liver function tests (LFTs) and a biochemical hyperthyroidism. Urinalysis will show a ketonuria.

Urine MCS should be performed to rule out a urinary tract infection (UTI).

Pelvic ultrasonography will rule out twin gestation or molar pregnancy and also adnexal masses.

Treatment

Admission to hospital is needed for any patient unable to maintain adequate hydration, weight loss or ketonuria.

Intravenous hydration with physiological (0.9%) saline or Hartmann's or Ringer's solution should be given. Double-strength saline should not be used because rapid correction of hyponatraemia may cause central pontine myelinolysis. Solutions containing dextrose should not be used because they do not contain enough sodium.

Antiemetics should be given. Phenothiazines are often used but the side effects are cumulative if combinations are used. Metoclopramide is often used.

Routine thiamine therapy should be given to prevent Wernicke's encephalopathy.

Thromboprophylaxis in the form of heparin must be given because dehydration is a risk factor for VTE (venous thromboembolism).

Steroids may be used in severe cases of hyperemesis unresponsive to usual treatment regimens.

Parenteral nutrition is sometimes needed for refractory cases.

TOP may be the treatment for severe illness causing significant maternal morbidity.

Essay 16

Discuss the epidemiology of gynaecological cancers and how to reduce their incidences.

Essay tips

- Discuss: give an account of cancers.

- Epidemiology: which age group affected by which cancer, associated risk factors.

- Gynaecological cancers: vulva, vagina, cervix, endometrium and ovaries.

- Measures to reduce them: screening, early diagnosis, treatment and follow-ups.

Essay plan

- cervix

- epidemiology/reduce incidence

- endometrium

- epidemiology/reduce incidence

- ovary

- epidemiology/reduce incidence

- vulva/vagina.

Specimen essay (336 words)

Gynaecological malignancies contribute significantly to mortality rates worldwide. Certain measures can be done to reduce the incidence and death from the diseases.

Cervical cancer is the second most common cancer in women. It is found in younger women, with HPV oncogenic subtypes 16 and 18 being strongly associated. Smoking, multiple sexual partners and sex under the age of 16 are risk factors.

Cervical screening using repeated Papanicolaou's smears has reduced the incidence of and deaths from this disease. The use of colposcopy and biopsies can help in rapid diagnoses and early treatment.

HPV immunisation may lead to a decrease in cervical cancer in the future.

Endometrial cancer usually occurs in postmenopausal women. Risk factors include obesity, late menopause and unopposed oestrogen therapy. Most cancers present early and have a good prognosis.

Screening measures have not been shown to be effective. Early detection with prompt referral of cases of postmenopausal bleeding and endometrial biopsies leads to prompt treatment.

Ovarian cancer is rare under the age of 30. It presents late, leading to a poor prognosis. There is a genetic predisposition. Patients with breast cancer (*BRCA*)-*1* gene mutations have a 40–60% lifetime risk of developing ovarian cancer; those with *BRCA-2* have a lower risk of 10–20%. High parity and the use of the COCP for 10–15 years reduce the risk of developing ovarian cancer.

Prophylactic bilateral oophorectomy may be offered to those with genetic abnormalities.

The use of ultrasonography and CA-125 as a screening tool for ovarian cancer is still at the research stage.

Vaginal and vulval cancers are rare and affect mainly elderly women. Women with a previous history of other anogenital cancers are at higher risk of developing vaginal and vulval cancers. HPV infection and smoking are associated with vaginal and vulval cancers. In utero exposure to diethylstilbestrol has been associated with clear cell adenocarcinoma of the vagina.

Measures such as stopping smoking can reduce the incidence of these cancers. Close vulvoscopic follow-ups with biopsies on those exposed to diethylstilbestrol are recommended on an annual basis.

Obstetrics

Essay 17

A 23-year-old primigravid woman has a scan at 30 weeks' gestation, which shows severe intrauterine growth restriction (IUGR). Discuss your further management.

Essay tips

The key words in this question are:

- 23-year-old woman/primigravida

- 30 weeks' gestation

- severe IUGR.

Essay plan

- History:

    – smoking, alcohol, drug abuse

    – underlying illness, pre-eclamptic toxaemia (PET), infection.

- Examination:

    – symphyseal fundal height, blood pressure (BP) and presentation

- Special investigations:

    – PET bloods, TORCH (toxoplasmosis, rubella, cytomegalovirus and herpes) screen

    – urine for microscopy, culture and sensitivity, protein

    – scan: repeat FAS, amniocentesis, CVS or FBS for karyotype

    – Doppler, biophysical profile (BPP), CTG (cardiotocography)

    – scan: estimated fetal weight (EFW), presentation, liquor, placenta, single umbilical artery.

- Management:

    – conservative (baby still growing, Doppler, CTG are normal), steroids/observations

    – IOL: severe fetal abnormality, no evidence of growth, Doppler/ CTG normal

    – Caesarean: abnormal Doppler/CTG no growth with non-cephalic presentation.

Specimen essay (339 words)

Maternal history factors include smoking, alcohol and drug use, and the woman's racial background. Pre-existing medical disorders may be present, eg renal or collagen disease, and pregnancy-related problems, eg pre-eclampsia. A history of infection and antiphospholipid antibody should be explored.

The 'fetal history' starts by checking dates and the results of a triple test and fetal anomaly scan. Multiple pregnancies should be excluded.

A general and obstetric examination should be performed, noting the symphyseal fundal height, maternal blood pressure, urinalysis and fetal presentation.

Maternal investigations should include an FBC, U&Es, LFTs, uric acid and coagulation screen if the blood pressure is elevated and a TORCH screen.

Investigation of the fetus includes a detailed ultrasound scan determining biparietal diameter (BPD) and abdominal circumference, with liquor volume determined and placental site noted, as well as a repeat fetal anomaly scan. Growth can be assessed by two scans more than 2 weeks apart.

Amniocentesis, or fetal blood sampling, may be performed to determine the karyotype if dysmorphic features are suspected.

Doppler studies of the umbilical, middle cerebral artery and the ductus venosus carried out to assist in the timing of delivery. CTG is also useful.

Management involving referral to a tertiary centre may be necessary. The parents should be closely involved in decisions. The balance here is between surveillance, with the attendant risk of intrauterine death, and the delivery of a preterm, compromised fetus

Admission of the mother and reduction of risk factors (smoking, alcohol and drug abuse, etc) may be required. Steroids in the form of betamethasone (12 mg daily for 2 days) should be administered to enhance fetal lung maturation.

Expectant management could be applied in a chromosomally abnormal fetus, a genetically small fetus or where Doppler and CTG assessments are satisfactory.

Delivery by Caesarean section is indicated in cases of severe oligohydramnios associated with absent or reversed end-diastolic flow or severe intercurrent maternal illness.

Induction of labour may be indicated when there is a severe (fatal) fetal abnormality or where there is a normal Doppler and no fetal growth.

Essay 18

Discuss the impact of prepregnancy clinics on future obstetric outcome.

Essay tips

The key words in this question are:

- discuss (pros and cons – have they made a difference?)

- prepregnancy clinics

- obstetric outcome.

Essay plan

- diabetes

- genetic disease

- chronic medical disorder, eg hypertension and medication

- previous obstetric problems, eg pre-eclampsia, abruptio placenta

- obstetric outcome.

Specimen essay (369 words)

Prepregnancy clinics make the earliest possible attempt to reduce maternal and perinatal morbidity and mortality. Ideally, both partners should be involved.

General measures should include ensuring/advising: optimal body weight; cessation of smoking and recreational drugs/substances, including alcohol; immunity to rubella; up-to-date cervical smear; and folic acid supplementation, with the higher dose given to women on anticonvulsant drugs and those with a previous child affected by a neural tube defect.

Information on teratogenic drugs should be given.

Women with diabetes are encouraged to attend prepregnancy counselling to normalise their Hb A_{1c} levels and optimise treatment for hypertension, retinopathy and nephropathy before pregnancy. This input is associated with a reduction in miscarriage and fetal abnormality rates. If an ACE (angiotensin-converting enzyme) inhibitor is used for nephropathy it should be changed before conception or in early pregnancy.

Genetic counselling is needed for couples known to have familial diseases or a previous handicapped child to learn about the risk to their offspring. Recurrence risks can be estimated and preimplantation diagnosis or invasive testing offered. This might be preceded by non-invasive tests such as nuchal translucency. The overall objective of these interventions is to prevent or detect the transmission of genetic disorders early and to offer termination of pregnancy if this is the wish of the couple. Women with previous PET (10–15%recurrence) or abruptio placenta (10% recurrence) should receive explanation of recurrence risks to enable her to plan any future pregnancies.

Women with a medical history could undergo a thorough assessment of their disease status, and a pregnancy planned for conception during a disease-free interval, eg systemic lupus.

Drug regimens could be adjusted to reduce/prevent the risk of fetal malformations, eg monotherapy in women with epilepsy. Advice against pregnancy and appropriate contraception might be given, eg to women with severe cardiac disease to reduce their risk of maternal morbidity and mortality.

Warfarin-treated women could be seen and the drug changed to low-molecular-weight heparin before pregnancy because warfarin is associated with embryopathy.

Psychiatric assessment of women with a history may be arranged and reassurance given about the teratogenicity of their drugs. A social network may be set up well in advance, involving the community psychiatric nurse, the GP and social worker, to support the couple during and after pregnancy.

Essay 19

Describe the management of a patient with chronic renal failure at 10 weeks' gestation.

Essay tips

- Describe what you would normally do in the clinic.

- Chronic renal failure: maternal and fetal risks, effects of pregnancy on disease progression.

- Ten weeks' gestation: cover the whole pregnancy.

- Management (not diagnosis): history, examination, investigations and treatments.

Essay plan

- First trimester: origin of problem/screening/ultrasonography.

- Second trimester: monitor renal function, fetal anatomy, ultrasonography, screening.

- Third trimester: real function, growth, delivery.

Specimen essay (291 words)

Chronic renal failure is associated with adverse maternal and fetal outcomes. The fetal risks include miscarriage, IUGR, preterm delivery and fetal death. Maternal complications include a decline in renal function, worsening proteinuria and hypertension during pregnancy.

First trimester

The origin of the renal failure may be the result of a genetic disorder such as polycystic kidney disease, which is an autosomal dominant condition with a 50% chance of affected offspring. Elicit whether she is on any form of dialysis. Dialysis treatment should continue.

The general condition of the patient should be checked and check the pulse and BP. On abdominal examination, check for masses and renal angle tenderness.

Urinalysis must be done and an MSU sample sent for microscopy, culture and sensitivity. Routine booking of bloods plus U&Es, serum creatinine and 24-hour protein excretion should be carried out.

BP control should continue with safe antihypertensives, eg labetolol or nifedipine.

Consider low-dose aspirin because the risk of pre-eclampsia is high. Patients should be seen regularly.

Renal physicians should be closely involved.

A dating ultrasound scan will also confirm fetal viability.

Second/third trimester

Offer second trimester serum screening for chromosomal abnormalities. Fetal anatomy ultrasonography at 20 weeks' gestation should be arranged.

At each visit send a urine sample for microscopy, culture and sensitivity because UTIs are common. Measure BP and treat hypertension as in any other hypertensive patient.

Regular assessment of renal function by creatinine clearance, 24-hour protein excretion, serum creatinine and urea is crucial.

Regular fetal monitoring with ultrasonography for growth, liquor volume and umbilical artery Doppler is essential because there is a risk of IUGR.

Delivery may be preterm as a result of worsening proteinuria, hypertension or renal function. Aim for vaginal delivery and reserve a Caesarean section for obstetric reasons.

Post partum

Monitor renal function and offer contraception.

Essay 20

A 32-year-old woman attends the antenatal clinic. She is known to be HIV positive. She is now 14 weeks' pregnant and wishes to discuss the implications of HIV in pregnancy. How would you counsel her?

Essay tips

The key words in this question are:

- 14 weeks' pregnant

- wishes to discuss

- implications of HIV in pregnancy

- how would you counsel her?

Essay plan

- antenatal: 14 weeks' pregnant

- fetal abnormality: TOP?

- HAART (highly active antiviral therapy) (teratogenesis)

- delivery: vertical transmission – labour/delivery

- postnatal: breast-feeding/neonatal treatment

- maternal prognosis.

Specimen essay (374 words)

A senior member of staff should counsel this woman and her partner in an atmosphere of privacy in a non-judgemental manner with time allocated for it.

The history of the stage of the disease, CD4 count and viral load should be obtained because high viral loads and low CD4 counts increase the risk of transmission.

If her partner is unaware of her infection she should be encouraged to tell him.

Markers of disease progression in the mother are not adversely affected by pregnancy and the maternal prognosis is unchanged.

Termination of the pregnancy needs to be discussed because of concerns for the unborn child and her own perceived reduced life expectancy.

The vertical transmission rate to the fetus is about 15%; this can be lowered to about 1–2% with a package of interventions including antenatal antiretroviral medication, elective Caesarean section, bottle-feeding rather than breast-feeding, and neonatal antiretroviral agents.

Higher transmission rates are found in patients with high viral loads, P24 antigenaemia, low CD4 counts ($< 200/ml$) and in premature deliveries < 34 weeks.

Highly active antiretroviral therapy (HAART) can reduce her viral load to undetectable levels and there is a negligible risk of vertical transmission to the fetus. There is some suggestion that an elective Caesarean section may not offer additional benefit for the fetus and vaginal delivery in this situation is best agreed on an individual patient basis.

Invasive prenatal diagnosis should be avoided, and detailed ultrasound-based screening used. There are no practical methods of prenatal diagnosis to predict which infants are or will be infected. Most neonatal infections occur during the perinatal period, which is the justification for the Caesarean section.

Neonatal HIV diagnosis is now being overcome by the introduction of DNA amplification testing such as PCR (polymerase chain reaction), rather than reliance on antibody assays. Maternal antibodies are unhelpful in fetal diagnosis.

Azidothymidine (AZT, zidovudine) is the only antiretroviral agent licensed for use during pregnancy in the UK. It has a relatively long track record of use in the perinatal period and carries a small risk of neonatal mitochondrial dysfunction. There are no long-term safety data on infants and children exposed to other antiretroviral agents.

Essay 21

A 26-year-old primigravida is admitted at 27 weeks' gestation, semi-conscious and with a history of convulsions. Outline the possible causes and principles of management.

Essay tips

The key words in this question are:

- 26-year-old primigravida
- admitted semi-conscious (therefore no history)
- 27 weeks' gestation
- outline
- possible causes
- principles of management.

Essay plan

- Pregnancy-related causes include:
  - eclampsia.
- Unrelated to pregnancy are:
  - cerebral vein thrombosis (CVT), cerebral infarction
  - thrombotic thrombocytopenic purpura (TTP)
  - drug and alcohol withdrawal
  - metabolic causes
  - epilepsy.
- Resuscitation A, B, C
- Communication
- Monitoring: maternal BP, oxygen saturation, urine output – fetal CTG.
- Investigation – FBC, clotting, BCP, ? CT/MRI, ? electroencephalogram (EEG).
- Treatment.

Specimen essay (368 words)

As in any obstetric emergency, the cause(s) may be related or unrelated to pregnancy. Principles of management include resuscitation, seizure control, stabilisation, investigation of cause and specific treatment.

Resuscitation of this semi-conscious patient begins with the appropriate positioning, clearance of the airway as needed and provision of an oxygen supply. Two large cannulas should be sited to secure venous access for fluid replacement and medications.

A multidisciplinary team approach involving senior obstetricians, anaesthetists, physicians, paediatricians, porters and haematologists should be assembled and a bed in the high-dependency unit (HDU) organised.

Vital signs should be monitored frequently, eg every 15–30 minutes initially, including blood pressure and pulse rate

A history from the patient herself, her notes, the referring healthcare worker, and her partner, family or friend should be extracted. The following are the important questions:

> Is this the first episode?
>
> Are any of following present: any prodromal symptoms, headache, restlessness, visual disturbance, a history of drug or alcohol abuse, diabetes, hypoadrenalism, hypopituitarism, liver failure, epilepsy or hypoparathyroidism?

A general and neurological examination should be performed, including a check for papillary oedema, neck stiffness and reflexes/clonus.

Investigations will include an FBC (including a platelet count and blood film for a differential count) and clotting screen, U&Es, LFTs, uric acid, blood glucose, calcium, sodium, drug levels as indicated and urinalysis. CT/MRI and EEG may be indicated and the fetal heart rate should also be monitored.

Treatment will depend on the underlying cause.

Eclampsia is treated with magnesium sulphate and antihypertensives. Steroids should be given and the infant delivered, regardless of its prematurity once the mother has been stabilised. Transport arrangements to a tertiary referral centre may be necessary.

Treatment of CVT is with anticonvulsants, as for epilepsy.

TTP can be treated with fresh-frozen plasma (FFP), and plasmapheresis and corticosteroids may be of benefit.

Drug and alcohol abuse is best treated in close liaison with the psychiatrist.

Patients with diabetes need a sliding scale for help in the correction of blood sugar levels. Hypoglycaemia may be corrected with glucagon in an emergency.

Other metabolic disorders can be corrected by delivery of the appropriate treatment through an infusion pump under close supervision and with the involvement of specialist physicians.

Essay 22

A 45-year-old grand-multiparous woman presents at 7 weeks' gestation in the antenatal booking clinic. Formulate a management plan specific to her pregnancy.

Essay tips

The key words in this question are:

- 45 years old – pregnant
- grand-multiparous
- 7 weeks' gestation
- formulate a management plan
- specific (note – related to grand multiparity and age).

Essay plan

- First trimester:
  - screening for Down's syndrome using nuchal translucency
  - ? CVS.
- Second trimester:
  - screening for Down's syndrome – fetal abnormality scan – growth scan ? IUGR
  - correct anaemia in pregnancy
- Third trimester:
  - fetal surveillance (USS , biparietal diameter, Doppler).
- Intrapartum:
  - ensure intravenous access, request an FBC and group and save.
  - partogram – the pelvic soft tissues may be more rigid as a result of the mother's age, and dystocia may occur.
- Post partum:
  - thromboprophylaxis, contraception.

Specimen essay (340 words)

Advanced maternal age and grand-multiparity combine to make this a high-risk pregnancy. Therefore consultant-led care is more appropriate.

First trimester

Routine booking investigations should be performed, eg haemoglobin level (? anaemia). Atypical antibodies are more common.

A medical, drug and obstetric history should be obtained because underlying medical disorders are more likely.

A booking scan to date the pregnancy is necessary.

The risk of Down's syndrome should be assessed (age-related risk is 1:50); a screening test (nuchal translucency or NT measurement) may be offered after counselling.

Invasive prenatal testing to establish the fetal karyotype may be requested if screening tests or history suggests.

Second trimester

Iron and folic acid supplementation may be needed throughout the pregnancy.

Hypertensive disorders and gestational diabetes are more common in older pregnant women; regular blood pressure and urine checks and a glucose tolerance test should be considered, especially if there is a glycosuria.

A fetal anomaly scan should be offered at 20–22 weeks' gestation.

IUGR is more common and close surveillance is required, including ultrasonography for fetal growth.

Third trimester and intrapartum

A placenta praevia should be excluded during the third trimester, especially if there is malposition or vaginal bleeding. There is a higher risk of a malpresentation and unstable lie of the fetus, necessitating admission towards term.

Spontaneous vaginal delivery should be anticipated, but a Caesarean delivery should be planned if there are other obstetric indications.

Thromboprophylaxis is indicated whether or not delivery is by Caesarean section.

In labour, a partogram should be used and, if required, the use of oxytocin should be sanctioned by a senior obstetrician, applied sparingly and with great caution because of the increased risk of uterine rupture.

The third stage of labour should be managed actively to reduce the risk of post partum haemorrhage (PPH), but an ergot-based preparation (eg Syntometrine) would be contraindicated in the presence of hypertensive disorders. Such women should be treated with 5 units Syntocinon.

Post partum

Contraception is needed during the postpartum period and, if necessary, continued social support organised for the mother and her family.

Essay 23

A multiparous woman, despite having good uterine contractions, remains in the second stage of labour for 2 hours. At pelvic examination the fetal head is found to be in the occipitotransverse position. Justify your decision on the mode of delivery.

Essay tips

The key words in this question are:

- multiparous

- good uterine contractions

- 2 hours in the second stage

- occipitotransverse position

- justify your decision

- mode of delivery.

Essay plan

- Caesarean

- vacuum

- manual rotation and forceps

- rotational forceps

- conservative – vaginal delivery.

Specimen essay (372 words)

Management of a delay in the second stage of labour in a parous woman should be handled or directly supervised by a senior obstetrician.

The past obstetric history should be obtained and further information gleaned from the clinical notes, especially relating to the modes of deliveries, sizes of the babies and their gestations at delivery.

An abdominal examination should be undertaken, to determine the degree of the fetal head engagement and to give a rough estimate of fetal size and state of the bladder. At pelvic examination, the capacity of the pelvis, the station of the fetal head, deflexion, presence and severity of caput, and moulding are all assessed. The time of the first stage and use of oxytocin and an epidural are useful.

Fetal well-being should be established by continuous CTG monitoring.

Expectant management is unlikely to lead to a normal vaginal delivery and poses several potential hazards for the mother, including uterine rupture.

Oxytocin in the presence of good uterine activity in a parous labour is inappropriate, and increases the risk of uterine rupture.

The options lie between an instrumental vaginal delivery and an emergency Caesarean section. Patient consent, transfer to theatre and appropriate analgesia given by a senior anaesthetist are all essential

Rotation of the head and vaginal delivery may be attempted in a non-distressed fetus with the vertex at or below the ischial spines and without significant caput and/or moulding. Manual rotation and a low cavity forceps delivery are an alternative.

A posterior metal vacuum cup may also be applied and autorotation achieved during traction. However, metal cups are associated with more scalp injuries.

The Kielland forceps, in experienced hands, may be used to rotate and complete delivery of the infant. There is, however, a higher risk of maternal genital tract trauma and post partum haemorrhage.

An emergency caesarean section should be undertaken if there are signs of obstruction, eg more than a fifth of the fetal head is palpable per abdomen and/or the vertex is above the level of the ischial spines, and where there is significant caput, moulding and deflexion of the fetal head. Caesarean section under these circumstances is hazardous, with risks of injury to the bladder, postpartum haemorrhage, lower segment tears, infection and thromboembolism postoperatively.

Essay 24

Compare and contrast the different drugs available for thromboprophylaxis in pregnancy.

Essay tips

The key words in this question are:

- compare and contrast (similarities and differences)

- different drugs

- available

- thromboprophylaxis in pregnancy.

Essay plan

- Routes of administration.

- Maternal side effects.

- Teratogenicity/fetal side effects.

- The need to monitor clotting parameters.

- Reversibility.

- These need to be considered at the following stages with the following drugs:

    - antenatal, intrapartum and post partum

    - aspirin

    - warfarin

    - heparin

    - LMWH

    - dextran.

Specimen essay (363 words)

Aspirin can be administered orally in a once-daily dose of 75 mg. The results of randomised trials have shown it to be effective in reducing the risk of thrombosis in medical and surgical patients, but the evidence for its efficacy in pregnancy is less robust. However, it has been shown to be safe with no risk of teratogenicity; nor is there any need to monitor blood levels. The risk of maternal gastrointestinal bleeding is very small. Its place is in the prevention of antenatal thromboembolism in women at low risk.

Heparin has to be administered via subcutaneous injection and compliance may be a problem. It has the advantage of not crossing the placenta and therefore has no adverse effects on the fetus. However, thrombocytopenia, especially the idiosyncratic immune-mediated variety occurring 6–10 days after the start of prophylaxis, is rare but potentially life threatening. Initial weekly platelet counts are recommended. Osteoporosis is another side effect, especially with long-term heparin use.

LMWH has a higher bioavailability and potentially better side-effect profile than unfractionated heparin, and can therefore be given once daily. High-risk women, eg those with thrombophilia, a family history of thromboembolism or recurrent thromboembolism in the current pregnancy, receive LMWH antenatally. Its drug effect can be speedily reversed if needed by protamine sulphate. LMWH can also cause osteoporosis and thrombocytopenia but less frequently than with heparin.

Warfarin can be given orally but it crosses the placenta and has a teratogenic risk of 5%. It should be avoided in the first trimester altogether, and may cause microcephaly and neurological abnormalities in fetuses exposed during the second trimester. Beyond 36 weeks' gestation, both retroplacental bleeding and intracerebral bleeding are reported. Close monitoring of the INR (international normalised ratio) is necessary and the effects can be reversed by the administration of FFP or vitamin K. Use during the antenatal period is restricted to women with metal heart valves whose thromboembolic risk is high. However, warfarin can be used for postnatal prophylaxis for women in all risk categories. There is a small amount secreted in the breast milk.

Dextran has been used in the past, but it interferes with maternal blood grouping and has therefore been abandoned.

Essay 25

Describe the complications of Caesarean section and discuss the possible methods of prevention.

Essay tips

The key words in this question are:

- describe

- complications

- Caesarean section

- discuss

- methods of prevention.

Essay plan

- Haemorrhage: case selection – senior input – technique.

- Infection: wound – endometritis.

- Thromboembolism mobilisation: drugs – TED (thromboembolism deterrent stockings).

- Surgical technique: gentle tissue handling – drainage – haemostasis.

Specimen essay (325 words)

The complications of Caesarean section may be avoided by the early recognition of risk factors. The appropriateness of Caesarean section delivery needs to be assured in the first instance

Haemorrhage might occur intra-operatively or postoperatively. Haemorrhage can be minimised by 'rubbing up' the uterus and an oxytocin infusion. Operations for placenta praevia should lead to precautions to prevent the massive haemorrhage and its complications, including crossmatching blood and ensuring the presence of a senior obstetrician and anaesthetist. This also applies to patients with a previous postpartum haemorrhage, obesity, prolonged second stage labour, pre-eclampsia or amnionitis, and when a classic Caesarean section is anticipated. In some circumstances, hysterectomy may be anticipated and the surgeon should be familiar with the variety of techniques to avoid this, eg a B-Lynch brace suture.

Exteriorisation of the uterus for repair has been shown to reduce blood loss in some studies but is not recommended by the National Institute for Health and Clinical Excellence (NICE).

Postoperative infection (endometritis) can be reduced by routine, prophylactic, broad-spectrum antibiotics.

UTIs can be minimised by aseptic catheter technique and prompt removal.

Bowel and bladder damage can be minimised by the careful identification of structures and tissues.

Wound infection and breakdown can be reduced by good surgical technique; secure haemostasis and wound drainage all help. The rectus sheath should be closed with large bites, using robust suture materials. For patients at high risk of postoperative dehiscence, mass closure using the Smeade–Jones technique and polydioxanone suture (PDS) material should be considered.

Bowel sounds return quicker with less infectious morbidity when non-closure of the peritoneum is undertaken.

Thromboembolism risk assessment for all women, followed by appropriate prophylaxis, including the use of TED stockings and LMWH, is mandatory.

Early mobilisation and discharge of women with straightforward operations may help to avoid nosocomial infections and reduce thromboembolism.

Protocols and guidelines should be available to prevent complications at Caesarean section, and regular audit and re-audit performed to ensure that high standards are continuously maintained.

Essay 26

A 29-year-old primigravid woman presents at 28 weeks' gestation with a marked oligohydramnios. Justify your investigations.

Essay tips

The key words in this question are:

- 29-year-old

- primigravid

- marked oligohydramnios

- justify

- investigations.

Essay plan

- maternal: smoking, drugs, PET, PPROM (premature prelabour rupture of membranes)

- fetal: abnormalities, IUGR, intrauterine device (IUD)

- placental: insufficiency

- vaginal examination

- ultrasonography

- Doppler

- CTG

- BPP

- cordocentesis.

Specimen essay (340 words)

Marked oligohydramnios describes the situation whereby the largest vertical pocket of amniotic fluid is considerably < 2 cm. It is associated with a 40-fold increase in the perinatal mortality rate. The causes may be maternal, fetal or placental.

Heavy smoking and prescribed drugs that may reduce the amniotic fluid volume (eg indometacin) should be explored in the history.

A speculum vaginal examination should be performed for the presence of amniotic fluid. The use of the nitrazine pH-based test for amniotic fluid may be used. The fern test may give a false negative at this stage of gestation.

The BP should be checked and an MSU obtained to check for the presence of protein. If positive, a 24-hour urine collection for total protein excretion should be started, and blood taken for an FBC, clotting screen, U&Es, urate and LFTs because severe PET might be a cause of the oligohydramnios.

Doppler waveform analysis of the umbilical artery will evaluate placental causes of oligohydramnios. In cases of absent or reversed flow, delivery may be indicated despite the early gestational age.

For the ultrasound diagnosis of IUGR, measurements of the head circumference biparietal diameter, abdominal circumference and femur length should be obtained, and the head-sparing effect would support the diagnosis. Doppler waveform analysis of the middle cerebral artery and a CTG would give some additional information. Some 70% of cases of marked oligohydramnios may be the result of IUGR.

A fetal blood sample may be obtained for karyotyping and analysis of fetal acid–base status, although there is a finite risk of fetal loss associated.

Ultrasonography to check for fetal viability and to exclude an underlying fetal abnormality. Emphasis should be placed on renal tract agenesis, of which Potter's syndrome is the most common. Lower urinary tract obstructions/abnormalities and hypoplasia of fetal lungs are other differentials.

Amniocentesis or CVS should be offered if there are features suggestive of clinical syndromes to establish the fetal karyotype. This may help to determine the management of the rest of the pregnancy.

Essay 27

A woman has had a failed trial of rotational forceps delivery and is now prepared to be delivered by emergency Caesarean section. Give a detailed account of the measures that you would implement to ensure a safe delivery.

Essay tips

The key words in this question are:

- the scenario as written in the first sentence

- give a detailed account

- measures (medical and surgical)

- you (ie don't hand over to the consultant).

Essay plan

- Preoperative:

  - disimpact head

  - catheterise

  - suitable analgesia.

- Intraoperative:

  - incision

  - push up head vaginally

  - inspect lower segment for tears

  - antibiotics/oxytocics.

- Postoperative:

  - anticoagulants/mobilise/speculum

  - counselling.

Specimen essay (308 words)

A second-stage Caesarean section after failed instrumental delivery is a potentially difficult procedure. Consent must be taken, and paediatricians and anaesthetists informed.

The supine position on the table with a slight, left-lateral tilt should be used.

Adequate analgesia (epidural or spinal) is needed if not already in place.

Manual disimpaction of a deeply impacted fetal head can be performed preoperatively.

An indwelling Foley catheter should be inserted before starting the procedure.

A large enough skin incision should be performed to create enough space.

Manual pressure from an extra person is sometimes required to push the deeply impacted fetal head up from the vagina, thereby facilitating delivery.

To decrease haemorrhage from the vagina, a high enough incision should be performed into the lower segment, avoiding cervical and vaginal tissues. A smile-shaped uterotomy is done and manually extended to guide potential tears upwards into the uterus rather than the broad ligament.

Rotation of the head to the occipitoanterior position not only eases delivery but also prevents tears into the broad ligament and vagina.

Controlled cord traction rather than manual removal of the placenta should be employed and the uterine cavity emptied of any residual placental tissue.

A contraction can be rubbed up by the assistant while the surgeon swiftly identifies and secures the angles of the uterotomy.

Intravenous oxytocin 20 units/l infusion should be started after delivery and continued for 6 hours.

Exteriorisation of the uterus is helpful to identify the full length of the incision and also to repair broad ligament and lower segment tears.

Prophylactic antibiotics should be given during the procedure.

A Sim's speculum examination should be performed at the end to identify and repair any trauma to the lower birth canal.

Postoperatively, prophylactic anticoagulants should be given in the form of LMWH.

Clear documentation is vitally important and counselling to explain the procedure to the woman.

Essay 28

A 33-year-old woman has had two second trimester losses in the past. She is now 13 weeks' pregnant and requests cervical cerclage. Would you support her request?

Essay tips

The key words in this question are:

- two second trimester miscarriages (maybe other pregnancies)

- 13 weeks' pregnant – requests cerclage

- would you support her request?

Essay plan

- ? Other pregnancies – first trimester loss/preterm labour/term deliveries.

- Specific to these second trimester losses:

    – ? painless/? preceded by rupture of membranes.

- Investigation results:

    – parenteral and fetal karyotyping

    – maternal thrombophilia screen

    – known uterine abnormality

    – vaginal swab results.

- ? Previous cerclage, ? connective tissue disorder.

- Alternatives?

- Transvaginal scans.

- Transabdominal cerclage.

Specimen essay (312 words)

Careful counselling of this woman and her partner is necessary to reach a sensible decision.

History

First trimester losses (TOP or miscarriage), preterm labours and term deliveries should be documented.

Painless pregnancy losses preceded by premature rupture of membranes would support the diagnosis of cervical incompetence.

Results of investigations enquired into, such as parenteral and fetal karyotyping, a maternal thrombophilia screen and vaginal swab results and postmortem reports.

A uterine anomaly, previous cervical surgery or connective tissue disorder necessitating different treatment options is important.

Counselling

A balanced discussion of the potential benefits and drawbacks of cervical cerclage and include possible alternatives.

Cerclage is treatment for cervical incompetence but its diagnosis is one of exclusion. Overall, 25 cerclages need to be performed to prevent one preterm birth. On the other hand, this woman's risk of a preterm birth with two second trimester losses is 15–20%. The Medical Research Council (MRC)/RCOG trial has also shown an improved neonatal outcome in terms of delivery after both 33 and 37 weeks' gestation.

It is also worthwhile to mention the procedure-related risk of pregnancy loss.

In women with a known uterine abnormality or connective tissue disorder a cerclage would be indicated.

Transabdominal cerclage has a success rate of 85–93%, but is obviously more invasive because it involves a laparotomy. Delivery would be by elective Caesarean section. However, if this woman has no living children and/or a previously failed vaginal approach, transabdominal cerclage may still be an option.

Transvaginal scanning could be offered to assess the cervical length and also to look for the feature of funnelling. The procedure has the advantage of being minimally invasive and can be repeated at any time.

Cerclage for asymptomatic cervical shortening to prevent prematurity is not proven.

Non-surgical alternatives would be progestogen vaginal pessaries.

Throughout the counselling session, the couple's views and aspirations need to be taken into consideration at all times.

Essay 29

Describe the management of a patient with acute fatty liver at 32 weeks' gestation.

Essay tips

- Describe: give an account of your care.

- Acute fatty liver is a serious condition.

- Management: history, examination, investigations and treatment.

Essay plan

- Stabilise and deliver

- Thirty-two weeks' gestation; preterm delivery, steroids, Caesarean section.

- Intensive therapy unit (ITU), liver specialists, anaesthetists, haematologists and paediatricians.

- Prognosis: poor if delayed diagnosis, good if prompt delivery.

Specimen essay (293 words)

Acute fatty liver is a rare but serious condition that can be lethal for both fetus and mother, especially is there is a delay in diagnosis.

A history of severe vomiting, bruising and bleeding may be present.

On examination the general condition of the patient, presence of jaundice, dehydration and signs of coagulopathy should be noted. Her pulse, temperature and BP should be checked. The abdomen must be checked for liver tenderness.

Investigations

An FBC, blood glucose levels, U&Es, LFTs and a clotting screen should be performed. In acute fatty liver there is profound hypoglycaemia and marked hyperuricaemia. Liver enzymes may be markedly raised. A liver biopsy is not recommended because there may be clotting defects. CT may reveal decreased attenuation suggestive of fatty infiltration.

A CTG for fetal well-being should be performed.

Treatment

Prompt delivery is the best treatment because this leads to improved outcomes for the fetus and mother. Give steroids for fetal lung maturation but these should not delay delivery which, at this gestation, would be by caesarean section.

Treat coagulopathy before the operation with FFP and vitamin K in collaboration with haematologists. Involve other specialists, eg paediatricians, liver specialists and anaesthetists.

Admission to the ITU with a multidisciplinary team input is needed.

Artificial ventilation may be needed if the patient is comatose.

Fulminant hepatic failure with multiple organ failure may occur, so close monitoring is needed and colonic emptying facilitated, eg nasogastric tube and enemas.

Neomycin should be given to reduce the intestinal production of ammonia and other infections aggressively treated, eg pneumonia or infections from catheters, lines.

Measures to reduce intestinal bleeding, eg antacids and H2-receptor blockers, should be given.

Prognosis: quick reversal of the clinical and laboratory findings follows delivery. Complete recovery with no long-term liver damage is usual.

Essay 30

A patient is 32 weeks' pregnant and has obstetric cholestasis. Describe your approach to her management.

Essay tips

- Thirty-two weeks: preterm, still some time for antenatal care.

- Obstetric cholestasis: definition, risks maternal/fetal.

- Describe: what will you do?

- Management: history, examination, investigations, treatment and follow-up.

Essay plan

- maternal surveillance

- FBC, LFT's, bile acids, hepatitis screen, coagulation screen, ultrasonography of gallbladder

- fetal surveillance

- CTG, Doppler, ultrasonography

- delivery mode/time

- Urosodeoxycholic acid

- recurrence rate, avoid COCP.

Specimen essay (298 words)

Obstetric cholestasis presents as itching in pregnancy without a rash. Its cause is not known. It can be associated with adverse fetal outcomes. It is a diagnosis of exclusion. Fetal risks include preterm delivery, intracranial haemorrhage and intrauterine death. Maternal risks are sleep deficiency and an increased risk of postpartum haemorrhage (PPH).

History

The severity of the itching is elicited. There may be a history of a similar episode in the last pregnancy. A history of dark urine, anorexia and fat malabsorption may be present.

On examination, excoriation and jaundice are important features to note.

The fundal height should be measured and the fetal heart listened to. The abdomen should be palpated for any liver tenderness.

Investigations

A CTG should be done to check for fetal well-being.

An ultrasound scan for fetal growth and liquor volume should be done.

Blood tests to include an FBC, LFTs and bile acids. The elevation of ALT (alanine transaminase) and bile acids may be found in this condition. A hepatitis screen should be performed

Treatment

Fetal surveillance with regular CTG monitoring is recommended because of a risk of intrauterine death, although the effectiveness of this strategy has not been proven.

Weekly LFTs and bile acids should be performed.

Vitamin K 10 mg orally daily should be given to reduce the risk of maternal and fetal bleeding.

Antihistamines may relieve itching.

Ursodeoxycholic acid 300 mg twice a day may relieve pruritis and improve LFTs and bile acids levels; however, it is not of proven benefit.

Delivery should be at 37–38 weeks' gestation but this strategy has not proved to reduce stillbirths.

Postdelivery, follow up with LFTs until they have returned to normal levels. Vitamin K should be given to the neonate.

The recurrence risk is 50% and COCPs should be avoided.

Essay 31

Discuss the causes and management of disseminated intravascular coagulation (DIC) in obstetrics.

Essay tips

- Discuss: means give an account.

- Causes of DIC: in obstetrics (take each cause one by one).

- Management: history, examination, investigations and treatment.

Essay plan

- abruptio placenta

- PET/HELLP

- septicaemia

- PPH

- amniotic fluid embolus.

Specimen essay (298 words)

DIC is a haematological disorder that can lead to massive haemorrhage. It has potential harmful results on the patient. The causes include massive haemorrhage such as from an abruption, pre-eclampsia/HELLP syndrome, amniotic fluid embolus, overwhelming infection and intrauterine death.

The diagnosis is made by evidence of a decrease in serum fibrinogen, platelets and elevated fibrin degradation products (FDPs), together with prolongation of the clotting parameters.

Treatment is by removal of the cause and replacement of blood products with blood (or packed cells), FFP, cryoprecipitate and platelet transfusions until the cause is adequately treated.

Abruptio placenta is a condition frequently associated with a rapid-onset DIC. The history is of a painful antepartum haemorrhage. An intrauterine death is common and the treatment is to correct the DIC with blood, FFP and cryoprecipitate, and then delivery of the fetus. PPH is common especially if the DIC is not fully corrected by the time of delivery.

PET/HELLP syndrome is a feature of pre-eclampsia with a reduced platelet count as a dominant feature and features of a DIC as a secondary aspect. Treatment is by delivery; transfusion of platelets and blood products is often not needed.

Amniotic fluid embolus usually causes a rapid severe DIC. The patient has vascular collapse and pulmonary oedema and a high maternal mortality. ITU treatment with ventilation, vascular support and blood replacement therapy is needed.

Septicaemia can cause a DIC from a variety of sources of the sepsis. The treatment is supportive with blood products, until the sepsis is treated by antibiotics and surgical drainage if necessary.

An intrauterine fetal death is an unusual cause of DIC in a chronic form; it may take more than 3 weeks to develop after an intrauterine death. Treatment is by replacement of blood and products followed by delivery of the fetus.

Essay 32

A 30-year-old woman arrives at a routine antenatal visit at 20 weeks' gestation smelling of alcohol. She admits to drinking excessively throughout pregnancy. Discuss your further management.

Essay tips

- excessive alcohol in pregnancy
- disclosure is too late for first trimester fetal problems
- issues relating to maternal health
- further management.

Essay plan

- history of alcohol intake/relevant other issues
- stigmata of alcoholic damage
- fetal status
- management/multiagency help/social support
- fetal growth
- delivery options.

Specimen essay (317 words)

The situation of a woman drinking heavily in pregnancy represents a risk to the woman, her existing children and the developing fetus.

Ascertainment of consumption is needed to assess the scale of the problem. Binge drinking is especially harmful. Other substances consumed or taken should be documented. Use of a dependence questionnaire (eg TACE) may help quantify the problem.

The social circumstances, especially partner and family support, and care arrangements for the existing children are important.

General examination of the woman is needed to look for hepatomegaly and signs of poor hygiene and self-neglect.

Biochemical markers of liver disease (especially γ-glutamyl transferase) renal disease and anaemia will assess target organ damage in the woman.

The fetal anatomy scan is important, because there may be damage to the fetus already, eg poor growth or structural abnormalities. The most important time for alcohol to cause a problem is between 4 and 10 weeks' gestation; however, alcohol-related problems can occur throughout pregnancy.

Follow-up scans in the third trimester are necessary to observe the growth pattern and liquor volume.

Referral to a specialist alcohol dependence team is essential to get help – medical, psychological and social – in order to reduce the intake of alcohol. Nutritional and vitamin supplementation may be needed.

Social Services involvement to safeguard the care of the existing children and the new baby is needed.

Detoxification programmes using benzodiazepines and phenobarbital could be offered if there is continued drinking and the request to stop.

Delivery options would depend on obstetric factors and evidence of fetal compromise by alcohol. Alcohol use in isolation would not indicate a caesarean section.

Examination of the newborn will establish the abnormal facial features (low-set ears, flattened philtrum, elongated mid-face) and small size associated with the fetal alcohol syndrome and other malformations.

Long-term paediatric involvement is needed because fetal alcohol syndrome is associated with neurodevelopmental delay and behavioural problems.

Contraception should be offered after delivery.

Objective Structured Clinical Examinations (OSCEs)

Station 1

Candidate instructions

Describe how you would conduct the vaginal delivery of an undiagnosed breech presentation discovered during the second stage of labour.

Examiner's mark sheet

1. The patient to start pushing when the cervix is fully dilated and the breech is visible at introitus.   [1 mark]

2. Would offer an elective episiotomy.   [1 mark]

3. If there were undue delay in descent, the candidate would consider inserting a finger in the baby's popliteal fossa to facilitate delivery of the legs.   [1 mark]

4. The candidate would rotate the sacrum anteriorly with the fingers on the anterosuperior iliac spine to avoid the soft abdomen.   [1 mark]

5. With the scapula in view, the candidate would rotate the baby 180° clockwise or anticlockwise (Lovsett).   [1 mark]

6. Would use finger to flex the cubital fossa in order to deliver the arms.   [1 mark]

7. The candidate explains why he or she would allow the breech to hang, without active traction.   [1 mark]

8. The delivery would be completed by applying a mid-cavity forceps to the after-coming head.   [1 mark]

9. If the head of a term baby gets stuck, the candidate would confirm that the cervix is fully dilated, apply suprapubic pressure to encourage flexion and complete the delivery with a pair of forceps. In extreme circumstances he or she would consider symphysiotomy, but realises that this is not usually advocated in the UK.   [1 mark]

10. If a preterm baby's head gets stuck, an incompletely dilated cervix is usually more likely, the candidate would consider cervical incisions at the 8 o'clock and 4 o'clock positions to avoid cervical branches of uterine vessels.   [1 mark]

Station 2

Candidate instructions

You are in a routine gynaecology outpatient clinic and have been asked to see a 32-year-old woman who has had lower abdominal pains for about a year.

She works in a factory and is living with her partner with whom she has one child, aged 6. You have the hospital notes, which indicate that she has been seen five times in the past 2 years in various clinics with symptoms of lower abdominal pain and backache. The diagnosis has not been established.

Role player's instructions

- You are a repeat hospital attender who is complaining of vague abdominal pains. There are no specific features of the pain; intercourse is painful but a different pain to the index problem.

- You are not happy with your relationship with your partner who works as a builder. He has a drinking problem and is violent towards you most weekends. He does not touch your child but has given you many bruises and cigarette burns.

- You have never said anything to your family and you live near to your partner's family with whom you get on.

- Disclose domestic violence only if asked by the doctor, eg 'Is everything alright at home?' or 'Is there a problem with your relationship?'. You can also disclose domestic violence if directly asked.

Examiner's mark sheet

1. Recognition of the issue of domestic violence.   [2 marks]

2. Polite, sensitive and non-judgemental attitude to patient when dealing with the issue of domestic violence.   [2 marks]

3. Establish if there is a risk to the well-being of the child.   [2 marks]

4. Establish if there is a threat of serious injury to the patient. Is it necessary for the woman to go to a woman's refuge?   [2 marks]

5. Offer referral to an outside agency, eg marriage guidance, woman's aid, police domestic violence team, GP.   [1 mark]

6. Offer contacts for treatment of partner's alcohol use, eg specialist alcohol agency, GP.   [1 mark]

Station 3

Candidate instructions

This woman has presented with a request for emergency contraception. Please take a history from her and outline a management plan.

Role player's instructions

- You are a 39-year-old woman who has never been married. You are not in a relationship but are sexually active on an intermittent basis.

- You work as a sales manager and your job entails frequent local and international travel. You had unprotected intercourse last night with a man whom you met at a party. You do not plan to see this man again. You do not use contraception but rely on condoms. Your menstrual cycle is usually regular. You have had two pregnancies resulting in two terminations of pregnancy in the past and do not plan to start a family in the near future. You have never had any illness in the past and have never undergone surgery.

- You are requesting emergency contraception.

Examiner's mark sheet

1. Taking a polite, sensitive, non-judgemental history with exploration of the sexual history and background of the patient, time since intercourse (< 72 hours) and time in menstrual cycle. [2 marks]

2. Pregnancy test and identification of the need for emergency contraception. [1 mark]

3. Outline of the different methods of emergency contraception available and their contraindications. [1 mark]

4. Hormonal (thromboembolism, hepatic disease, hypertension), intrauterine contraceptive device (IUCD), (pelvic inflammatory disease or PID, ectopic). [2 marks]

5. Explanation of suggested form of contraception; PC4 2 tablets each dose or levonorgestrel (Levonelle One Step) 1 tablet each dose, explanation of timing, vomiting (further treatment if vomits in 2 hours), effect on next period (may be late), abstinence or barrier methods for rest of cycle and need for a follow-up if no period is seen at end of cycle. [2 marks]

6. Future contraception: consider depo/implants/IUS . [1 mark]

7. Sexual health advice, screen for sexually transmitted infections (STIs)/ risks related to lifestyle/barrier contraception. [1 mark]

Station 4

Candidate instructions

Mrs Amanda Jones has booked at 14 weeks' gestation in her second pregnancy.

Her first ended in delivery at 39 weeks by emergency Caesarean section for fetal distress in labour. Her baby is 2 years old and healthy. Two weeks after delivery she had a major pulmonary embolus.

Would you please take a history from her and outline the plan of management for the pregnancy.

Role player's instructions

- You had a major pulmonary embolus after the last pregnancy and are worried about another. Your last pregnancy was in another town.

- You and your baby are now well but you do have one leg (the right) that is always larger than the other.

- You spent 2 days in the intensive care unit (ICU) and were treated afterwards for 6 months with warfarin tablets.

- The doctors told you that there was 'nothing abnormal with your blood tests' when you were tested for clotting disorders after you were better.

- Your mother died of a stroke when she was 42 and one of your sisters also had a 'clot in the leg' on two separate occasions.

- Your father is 56 and has mild angina and your older brother is well.

Questions to be asked

1. You would like to know what will happen in this pregnancy and whether you need treatment.

2. Could you have warfarin as you have had it in the past?

3. You would like an elective Caesarean. What will your management be with regard to any anticoagulation?

Examiner's mark sheet

1. Establish the validity of the history of pulmonary embolus (ICU and the 6 months of treatment with warfarin).   [2 marks]

2. Enquire about the thrombophilia screen result and offer to recheck if it cannot be found.   [2 marks]

3. Take a relevant family history and establish the correct facts. [2 marks]

4. Offer prophylactic anticoagulation with LMWH both antenatally and 6 weeks postnatally; explain the reasons for LMWH rather than warfarin, ie problems with warfarin (mid-trimester: optic atrophy, microcephaly; last trimester: fetal bleeding, retroplacental bleeding).   [2 marks]

5. Outline the peripartum management of anticoagulation, ie last injection 24 hours before the operation and recommence 4 hours after the spinal/epidural catheter removed.   [2 marks]

Station 5

Candidate instructions

You are asked to see a primiparous woman who has been admitted to the antenatal ward at 24 weeks' gestation with symptoms of early labour. The senior house officer (SHO) has already seen her and does not think that she is in premature labour.

The SHO tells you that the woman is agitated and restless; she is not very clean and her clothes are dirty. Taking a blood specimen has been difficult and after questioning about her arms the woman has disclosed intravenous heroin use to the SHO.

Role player's instructions

- You have booked in this pregnancy but did not disclose to the midwife or doctor that you have used heroin for about a year. Initially you were a light user but your use has been about £50 per day over the last month since you 'split up' with the baby's father.

- You have not shared needles or taken other drugs.

- You smoke 20 cigarettes/day and drink until you get drunk once or twice a week.

- Your family does not know of the drug use and you are ashamed to tell them.

- You now nominally live at home but often sleep at friends' places. You are unemployed at present.

- Finance for the heroin was from your partner originally, but recently you have been involved in prostitution.

- You are worried about harm to the baby and whether the baby will suffer from the addiction after birth.

Examiner's mark sheet

1. Non-judgemental questioning about her use of drugs covering: needle sharing, intravenous or smoking heroin, cost per day as an estimate of scale of use, other drug use, previous methadone/buprenorphine programme and neonatal withdrawal symptoms.   [3 marks]

2. Past medical history covering: STIs (need for screening), thrombophlebitis, groin/skin abscesses, hepatitis and HIV testing.   [1 mark]

3. Social circumstances must be questioned: living conditions, financial support and plans for child care/family involvement.   [1 mark]

4. Explanation that a methadone programme will be needed.   [1 mark]

5. Hepatitis screening should be offered if not already done and hepatitis B immunisation of mother and neonate should be offered.   [1 mark]

6. HIV testing should be offered if not already done.   [1 mark]

7. Screening for STIs should be offered.   [1 mark]

8. Need to explain social worker involvement.   [1 mark]

Station 6

Candidate instructions

There has been increased expenditure for prophylactic antibiotics at hysterectomy on the gynaecology ward. Describe in detail to the examiner how you would set up an audit for this.

Examiner's mark sheet

1. Define audit.   [1 mark]

2. The candidate is aware that the RCOG standard is to give prophylactic
    antibiotics to all patients undergoing hysterectomy (grade A
    evidence).   [2 marks]

3. The exact antibiotic, route and duration of use are contentious, but it
    should be broad spectrum with additional anaerobic cover.   [1 mark]

4. Candidate would liaise with the clinical director, audit department,
    pharmacy and ward sister to devise a data sheet and see whether
    local agreed practice or protocol meets the standard.   [2 marks]

5. Would collect data sheets or put data onto a computer and analyse it
    over a set period.   [1 mark]

6. Would analyse data to see how local practice compares with the
    existing standard and suggest changes or make recommendations.
                                                                           [1 mark]

7. Candidate would re-audit antibiotic practice after a set period of time
    from effecting the change to closing the loop.   [2 marks]

Station 7

Candidate instructions

Mr and Mrs Smith have been referred to you for counselling after Mrs Smith's 12-week ultrasound scan.
The 12-week scan report shows:

- *Monochorionic diamniotic twin pregnancy:*

  - *fetus 1: crown–rump length (CRL) 75 mm, fetal heart beat seen, nuchal translucency (NT) 22 mm*

  - *fetus 2: CRL 77 mm, fetal heart beat seen, NT 34 mm.*

In addition:

- *Age-related risk of Down's syndrome 1:652.*

- *Fetus 2 adjusted risk of Down's syndrome 1:123.*

Discuss with the examiner the specific counselling that you would give Mr and Mrs Smith and why.

Examiner's mark sheet

1. The candidate explains the need to know more about Mrs Smith's obstetric history (parity, previous aneuploidy, age, fertility and if this was a planned pregnancy).   [1 mark]

2. Explains what nuchal translucency is, counsels sensitively, keeps medical jargon to a minimum and gives facts and information. Reiterates that only when Mrs Smith has been fully informed of the options and risks can she make a decision – the decision is hers, not the doctor's.   [1 mark]

3. Although NT for fetus 1 is normal, for fetus 2 it is abnormally high, and therefore invasive testing would be offered.   [1 mark]

4. Invasive testing is an option but is not mandatory.   [1 mark]

5. The option of biochemical screening is not appropriate in twins.
                                                               [1 mark]

6. Both chorionic villus sampling (CVS) and amniocentesis are performed with a single-pass needle, and are used to determine the karyotype of both twins.   [1 mark]

7. The advantages and disadvantages of CVS versus amniocentesis.
                                                               [1 mark]

8. Even if the chromosome analysis is normal, there is still a small risk of cardiac abnormalities and other rare genetic syndromes.   [1 mark]

9. If chromosomal abnormalities are found, offer the option of termination of pregnancy (TOP).   [1 mark]

10. The need for further scans because of the risks associated with monochorionic twin pregnancies, including: preterm delivery, twin–twin transfusion syndrome and intrauterine growth retardation (IUGR).
                                                               [1 mark]

Station 8

Candidate instructions

Mr and Mrs Williams have come for the results of Mrs Williams's 20-week ultrasound scan.

The 20-week anomaly ultrasound scan report shows:

- *Mild ventriculomegaly, lumbosacral meningocele evident.*

- *Bilateral talipes.*

- *Liquor volume normal, fetal anatomy and biometry consistent with dates.*

Explain the significance of the ultrasound scan report to the examiner and say how you would counsel/advise the patient.

Examiner's mark sheet

1. Explains that a meningocele is an open neural tube defect and that it does not contain neural tissue, unlike a meningomyelocele, so the former has a better prognosis. [1 mark]

2. The lumbosacral region is the most common site; the lower the lesion, the better the prognosis. [1 mark]

3. Ventriculomegaly is often associated with lumbosacral spina bifida and can be associated with aneuploidy (consider amniocentesis), other central nervous system (CNS) defects and congenital infections. [1 mark]

4. Talipes is often associated with lumbosacral spina bifida and may respond to physiotherapy or surgery. [1 mark]

5. An affected child may have voiding difficulties in the long term. [1 mark]

6. The mother would be asked about her medical history, including whether she has ever had epilepsy, used periconceptual folic acid or had a previous pregnancy with a neural tube defect. [1 mark]

7. The candidate would tell the parents that they have the option to see a paediatrician/neurosurgeon to discuss the prognosis. [1 mark]

8. The candidate says that the option of terminating or continuing the pregnancy would be discussed with the parent(s). [1 mark]

9. The mode of delivery would be discussed with the parents – Caesarean section versus vaginal delivery – a lower segment Caesarean section (LSCS) would be offered, but the optimal route is debatable. [1 mark]

10. Discusses increasing the dose of folate to 5 mg daily for 12 weeks pre-pregnancy for future pregnancies, and requesting possible 16-week ultrasound scan. [1 mark]

Station 9

Candidate instructions

In this roleplay, you are required to take a relevant history from Mrs Jones who has been referred to you by the day assessment unit midwife with a blood pressure reading of 160/115 and 1+ proteinuria.

Indicate to the examiner the appropriate investigations that you may want to request (and why) and discuss possible treatment options with this 'patient'.

Role player's instructions

- You are 37 years of age and in your second pregnancy.
- Your first pregnancy was 7 years ago and resulted in a male infant delivered at 40 weeks by Caesarean section for failure to progress at 7 cm dilatation after being induced for pre-eclampsia.
- You are now 39 weeks' pregnant.
- This was an unplanned pregnancy and you are planning to give the child up for adoption after its birth.
- You are separated from your husband and this pregnancy is by another man.
- You have had a persistent frontal headache for the last 12 hours that is not settling.
- You are currently unemployed, and do not smoke, take drugs or drink alcohol.
- You have had no problems in the pregnancy until now.
- You are otherwise fit and well and have had no other operations or medical conditions of note; you take no medication and are not allergic to anything.
- The midwife has palpated your abdomen and, although baby is 'head down', she feels that you are small for dates.
- Ask the candidate if you can go home because you are keen to get back to your son.
- Ask the candidate if you and the baby will be all right.
- If possible, say you would like to avoid a Caesarean section this time.

Examiner's mark sheet

1   The candidate makes good eye contact, has good rapport, listens to
     the patient appropriately.   [1 mark]

2   Discusses the risks for pre-eclampsia (previous pre-eclampsia,
     different partner, age).   [1 mark]

3   Takes a general history.   [1 mark]

4   Admits the patient and requests appropriate investigations: mid-
     stream urine sample for culture; 24-hour urine collection for protein
     estimation; full blood count (FBC); urea and electrolytes (U&Es),
     including urate; liver function tests; and clotting times.   [2 marks]

5   Shows an appreciation of the pros and cons of treatment
     (antihypertensives/wait to see if BP settles).   [1 mark]

6   Is aware that induction of labour may be an option if the cervix is
     favourable, and is aware of the small (0.5–1%) risk of scar rupture
     from the previous Caesarean section. The candidate has considered
     using the Bishop score and artificial rupture of membranes instead of
     prostaglandin induction of labour.   [2 marks]

7   Discusses the option and pros/cons of a semi-elective/non-urgent
     Caesarean section.   [2 marks]

Station 10

Candidate instructions

Miss Peak, 23 years of age, has been referred to you by her GP with amenorrhoea for 6 months and galactorrhoea of 3 months' duration. Her serum prolactin level is 7600 IU.

Explain to the examiner those specific relevant features that you would want to elicit from her history, the relevant investigations that you may require and how you may manage her.

Examiner's mark sheet

1. History: could be pregnant, has recently been pregnant, has finished breast-feeding, on medication causing galactorrhoea, and check visual impairment, symptoms of thyroid disease. [2 marks]

2. Investigations: pregnancy test, serum prolactin, thyroid function tests, FSH/LH levels, pelvic ultrasound scan, skull radiographs and MRI/CT of the pituitary fossa. [3 marks]

3. Treatment: the examiner to say that all investigations are normal, except for a raised prolactin level and a pituitary adenoma. The examiner would ask the candidate how she or he would treat the patient:

    – carefully and simply explains the treatment options to the patient

    – would await the results of the pituitary scan,
    then:

    – if prolactin > 8000 IU and prolactinoma < 1 cm would treat with drugs (bromocriptine versus cabergoline)

    – if prolactin < 3000 IU and prolactinoma > 1 cm, says that surgical referral may be more appropriate, especially if visual disturbances are present. [3 marks]

4. The examiner asks the candidate how she or he would manage the patient if she is pregnant. The candidate should say that the prolactin level is difficult to monitor because it is raised in pregnancy, but the patient would need pituitary fossa imaging if her visual symptoms or headaches persist. Bromocriptine can be safely given and the mother can breast-feed. Says there is no need to alter the mode of delivery. [2 marks]

Station 11

Candidate instructions

Explain to the examiner how you would manage a case of postpartum haemorrhage. The examiner prompts you that the patient is still bleeding after each suggestion that you make.

Examiner's mark sheet

1. The candidate would assess the patient's airway, breathing, circulation; site two large-bore intravenous cannulae; take blood for an FBC, clotting, crossmatch (initially 4–6 units). Give fluids and blood when needed, and maintain a strict fluid–balance chart, central line and urinary catheter. As appropriate, would explain the situation to the patient and her partner, inform them of what steps she or he is taking and why. [2 marks]

2. The candidate would look for causes of the haemorrhage, and explains that in most cases this will be an atonic uterus. Says that they would evacuate clots, remove retained products/placenta if necessary and examine for cervical or vaginal tears. [1 mark]

3. Would make sure that the uterus is well contracted: manually rub up a contraction/apply bimanual pressure; give 5 IU oxytocin as an intravenous bolus and ergometrine 0.5 mg. [1 mark]

4. Would give carboprost intramuscularly, 250 μg every 15 min up to a maximum of eight doses. The candidate explains that, if the patient loses > 1.5 l of blood, the consultant obstetrician should be informed as well as the duty consultant haematologist and anaesthetist. [1 mark]

5. Would consider packing the uterus with gauze or gauze soaked in prostaglandin gel, misoprostol pessaries or intramyometrial carboprost. [1 mark]

6. A balloon tamponade using an intrauterine balloon catheter and vaginal pack may be highly effective. [1 mark]

7. Would consider radiological embolisation of the uterine arteries with a gelatine sponge. [1 mark]

8. Would consider a B-Lynch suture (if caused by uterine atony), ligation of uterine arteries or anterior division of the internal iliac arteries. [1 mark]

9. Would consider a subtotal hysterectomy with ovarian conservation if bleeding persists or haemorrhage becomes uncontrollable. [1 mark]

Station 12

Candidate instructions

Ms Duke is 38 years of age, nulliparous and HIV positive, with large bilateral hydrosalpinges. She, together with her female partner, wishes to have a baby in the very near future and wants to ask you some questions. Counsel her appropriately.

Examiner's mark sheet

1. Advises in vitro fertilisation (IVF) with donor sperm.   [1 mark]

2. Advises her that her age needs to be considered; IVF on the
    National Health Service (NHS) for women under 40 years of age is
    recommended.   [1 mark]

3. The severity of her HIV disease needs to be considered; check
    her CD4 count, viral load, antiretroviral therapy and acquired
    immunodeficiency disease (AIDS)-defining illnesses.   [1 mark]

4. The local infertility ethics committee (the IVF coordinator, holder of
    the HFEA [Human Fertilisation and Embryology Authority] licence,
    embryologist, counsellor and genitourinary medicine physicians) will
    need to be involved.   [1 mark]

5. Advises her of the need to consider the welfare of her unborn child
    – HIV transmission has a risk of 15–45%; also check her partner's
    status.   [1 mark]

6. She will need to give details of her general history, any convictions,
    any psychiatric history and her hepatitis B and C status. Her partner's
    demographics will also be needed.   [1 mark]

7. Although lesbian status is not a contraindication, it will need to be
    discussed by the ethics committee and can involve HFEA guidance.
                                                                   [1 mark]

8. The candidate says that they would advise bilateral tubal ligation
    because this gives a better implantation rate.   [1 mark]

9. Advises that, if pregnancy is achieved, she will need antiretroviral
    therapy during pregnancy and an elective Caesarean section; she will
    also need to bottle-feed to reduce the risk of vertical transmission to
    the baby to 2%.   [1 mark]

10. Risks of IVF: natural/short-/long-cycle regimens; superovulation with
    gonadotrophins; follicle tracking; time off work; the success rate of
    around 15%, depending on her age and the unit; the risks of ovarian
    hyperstimulation syndrome; ovarian accidents; multiple pregnancy;
    vertical transmission risk; and the long-term risk of ovarian cancer with
    superovulation.   [1 mark]

Station 13

Candidate instructions

Mrs Jones is 31 years of age and in her first pregnancy. She attended the booking clinic at 16 weeks' gestation and is now 18 weeks' pregnant. She is referred to you with the results of her booking blood test for rubella, and for a history of malaise, flu-like symptoms and a pinpoint macular rash that appeared 2 days ago. She did not receive rubella immunisation at school. The microbiology laboratory report shows:

- *rubella IgG = < 10 (non-immune)*

- *rubella IgM = positive.*

She would like to know the significance of the test result, the implications for her pregnancy and what her options are for this pregnancy.

Examiner's mark sheet

1. The candidate gives a simple explanation of what rubella is (a virus) and what the test results mean; says it is unlikely that they are the result of past exposure to rubella, but are probably the result of a recent exposure.   [1 mark]

2. Explains where the infection may have come from (contact), and the need to stay away from pregnant women for 8 days after the onset of the rubella rash.   [1 mark]

3. Although she has recently had rubella, it does not mean that her baby will invariably be infected or affected by it. The risks of congenital infection if exposure occurs at 16 weeks' gestation are: infection rate in fetuses about 50% and congenital defects present in about 50% of these.   [1 mark]

4. The rash usually occurs about 16 days after exposure to the rubella virus, so she was probably exposed to the virus at around 16 weeks' gestation.   [1 mark]

5. The need for follow-up in the fetal medicine centre or with a consultant virologist to discuss possible further investigations, including cordocentesis (to establish whether the fetus is infected), but the risk of miscarriage with such a procedure is about 2%.   [2 marks]

6. A TOP is an option.   [1 mark]

7. She does not need to be immunised because she will now have natural immunity.   [1 mark]

8. Fetal abnormalities may not be seen on ultrasonography (deafness, retinopathy, cataracts, mental handicap, hepatosplenomegaly).   [1 mark]

9. There is a risk of intrauterine death. Alternatively, the baby could be born with a handicap, in which case she would see a paediatrician to discuss the longer-term prognosis.   [1 mark]

Station 14

Candidate instructions

You are performing a total abdominal hysterectomy with ovarian conservation and you want to use diathermy for haemostasis. However, in spite of sustained pressure on the diathermy pedal, nothing happens. Explain what actions you would take and discuss the use of diathermy with the examiner.

Examiner's mark sheet

1. The candidate explains that they would first check that the machine was switched on, and the diathermy unit was properly connected to the machine and the patient pad (if monopolar). The candidate would check that the output settings were high enough to produce an effect and consider changing the lead if the problem persisted. Says that they would ensure that they were pressing on the diathermy pedal rather than on the cutting pedal.   [1 mark]

2. The differences between monopolar and bipolar settings: monopolar means that the current passes through the patient's body, and may result in a larger dissipation of heat energy compared with bipolar diathermy where the current acts between the two local electrodes.
                                                                   [2 marks]

3. The different forms of monopolar coagulation:

    – spray: delivers superficial, high voltage, is not in contact with tissue, and is good for use under water or for a diffused haemorrhage

    – fulguration: delivers high voltage with a good depth of coagulation to major bleeds

    – desiccation: produces a slow drying out of tissues with the electrode in contact with tissues; it is the most commonly used.   [1 mark]

4. Explains which modality they would use to cut through:

    – the skin: monopolar cutting diathermy with blend – for cutting and haemostasis without the need for a precise limit of heat damage to tissue

– the rectus sheath: monopolar cutting diathermy with blend – for cutting and haemostasis without the need for a precise limit of heat damage to tissue

– to obtain haemostasis at the ovarian pedicle: bipolar diathermy

– to obtain precise haemostasis and to limit heat damage to the surrounding tissues, eg to the ureter. [2 marks]

5. Explains which settings they would set the machine to. Says the exact value is unimportant, but a reasonable setting would be 35 diathermy and 35 cutting with blend. [1 mark]

6. Explains what they would do if they noticed a burning smell after closing the skin at the end of the procedure: candidate would check the leg pad on the patient for skin burns – check whether or not it was properly applied flush to the skin. If a skin burn were noticed, the candidate would fill out a risk-management form, inform the head theatre sister and consultant in charge of the case, ask the advice of a plastic surgeon and explain the incident to the patient. [2 marks]

7. Explains how the chances of injury could be minimised when using diathermy in gynaecological surgery:

– put the electrode in its holster between uses – do not leave the electrodes on the patient

– do not use high-voltage spray coagulation

– use low-voltage desiccation coagulation

– be aware of a direct coupling risk

– use a bipolar technique if possible

– always check the integrity of instruments/cable insulation of electrodes

– follow audit department guidelines on the use of diathermy

– discuss relevant issues with the departmental risk manager

– ensure that risk management forms/trigger response forms are filled out appropriately. [1 mark]

Station 15

Candidate instructions

You are asked to advise this young 18-year-old woman about her contraceptive options. Explain your advice to her.

Examiner's mark sheet

1. The candidate says that they would ask the patient: if she is in a relationship; when she had her last menstrual period; and if she has any salient medical conditions that may alter the advice given. [1 mark]

2. Explains the different types of temporary contraception:

    – hormonal – COCP, depo injection, implants, Mirena coil

    – barrier methods – condom, cap, diaphragm

    – intrauterine devices – copper and inert devices. [2 marks]

3. Explains the permanent methods of contraception, including sterilisation, and that this is not routinely recommended for such young women. [1 mark]

4. Advises 'double Dutch' contraception (ie protection from infections such as that caused by *Chlamydia* through the use of condoms and a reliable contraceptive method such as the pill or depo injection). [2 marks]

5. Advises on advantages and disadvantages of each option. [1 mark]

6. Asks her if she has any particular preferences. [2 marks]

7. Explains when the patient should seek emergency contraception. [1 mark]

Station 16

Candidate instructions

A 20-year-old pregnant woman with type 1 diabetes attends for her very first antenatal booking visit at 22 weeks' gestation. Explain how you would counsel her.

Examiner's mark sheet

1. Asks: if she has any other relevant history; other medical illnesses; takes other medications; parity; how long she has been diabetic for and what is her level of diabetic control; and if she has had any scans to confirm her dates.   [½ mark]

2. Explains that booking normally occurs earlier than 22 weeks. However, the candidate reassures her and explains the need to arrange various appointments.   [1 mark]

3. The candidate says that they would arrange a multidisciplinary (obstetrician or physician with an interest in obstetric medicine, diabetes nurse specialist, midwife, dietitian) clinic appointment to monitor blood glucose control closely (aim for preprandial levels < 6 and postprandial levels < 8 mmol/l – via home blood glucose monitoring). Explains that good blood glucose control will help the health of both the mother and the baby.   [1 mark]

4. The candidate would arrange booking blood tests (FBC, blood group and antibody check, syphilis serology, hepatitis B serology, HIV serology [with consent], renal function and glycated haemoglobin [Hb A_{1c}]) (for average blood sugars over the last 6–8 weeks). Obtain an MSU for microscopy, culture and sensitivity (as asymptomatic bacteriuria may be present) and bedside testing for microalbuminuria, suggestive of renal impairment, and arrange for an eye test.   [1 mark]

5. Would explain the need for an ultrasound scan if she has not had one, to estimate the gestational age (especially if she is uncertain of the date of her last menstrual period or her periods had been irregular); check for congenital anomalies, number of fetuses and location of the placenta. This is important because babies born to women with diabetes have a higher risk of congenital anomalies than those born to women who are not diabetic.   [1 mark]

6. It may be more difficult to screen for chromosomal anomalies at this gestation (too late for NT and at the maximum limit for serum biochemical screening). The candidate would counsel that 'soft markers' on ultrasonography may help to screen for chromosomal abnormalities, although they are not very sensitive or specific unless two or more are present, or opt for cordocentesis, but the risk of miscarriage with this would be at least 2%. [1 mark]

7. Explains the need for hospital-based and consultant-led care throughout the pregnancy (as she is in a higher risk group). [½ mark]

8. The candidate would arrange further tests for Hb A_{1c}, and serial scans to monitor fetal growth and amniotic fluid volume at around 28, 32 and 36 weeks' gestation (babies with diabetes may be macrosomic, have polyhydramnios or even exhibit IUGR). [1 mark]

9. Explains the risks of diabetic pregnancy: poor blood sugar control/ hypoglycaemia, retinopathy and renal dysfunction, macrosomia, shoulder dystocia, infections, preterm labour, high blood pressure, congenital anomalies, neonatal respiratory distress syndrome, neonatal hypoglycaemia, neonatal admission in the immediate postpartum period and the small increased risk of intrauterine death. Would reassure her that with close monitoring and appropriate management most diabetic pregnancies do not experience such complications. [1 mark]

10. Counsels her that she may consider induction of labour at 38–39 weeks' gestation (to avoid the risk of intrauterine death). [1 mark]

11. Explains that her insulin requirement is likely to increase, especially during the last trimester, and that postnatally this will return to her pre-pregnant levels. [½ mark]

12. Asks her if she has any questions or needs clarification on any of the points raised. [½ mark]

Station 17

Candidate instructions

A woman presents to you in the antenatal clinic at 17 weeks' gestation with an ultrasound scan report showing an increased nuchal fat pad of 45 mm in the fetus and no other anomalies. This is her first ultrasound scan. Explain how you would counsel her.

Examiner's mark sheet

1. The candidate explains the need to obtain a medical history, parity, previous history, whether she knows of any genetic/chromosomal problems in the family and if she has had serum biochemical screening, and check if there is any history of viral infections in this pregnancy. [1 mark]

2. Explains what the ultrasound scan has shown – an increased area of thickness in the soft tissue between the skin and the spine at the back of the baby's neck and that there are no other abnormalities seen. [1 mark]

3. Explains that most women have this scan between 11 and 14 weeks' gestation and the fluid behind the neck at this time is called 'nuchal translucency' (which all fetuses have to some degree and which disappears by 14 weeks in most cases). After 14 weeks' gestation, the presence of a sonolucent area may represent extra fluid that may be slowly resolving (nuchal translucency), be a sign of hydrops (fetal heart failure) or be an extra area of tissue that is a variant of normal. [1 mark]

4. Explains that such a finding may be associated with chromosomal abnormalities such as Down's syndrome or heart anomalies. In the absence of other markers, this is unlikely. Informs her that she would be referred to the local fetal medicine unit for risk assessment and possibly fetal echocardiography. [2 marks]

5. Such a finding may be a normal variant and there is every chance that the baby will be normal, although this cannot be guaranteed. One option would be to wait until the 20-week scan to check all the baby's anatomy. [1 mark]

6. Invasive testing (such as amniocentesis with a risk of miscarriage of 1%) would be diagnostic. [1 mark]

7. Counsels her that the risks of having an affected child need to be weighed against the risks of miscarriage, and that the fetal medicine unit is best qualified to give her the exact risks involved. [1 mark]

8. The neck thickness may become greater as the pregnancy progresses, but it usually regresses and is unlikely to be evident at birth. [1 mark]

9. Asks if she has any further questions that she would like answered. [1 mark]

Station 18

Candidate instructions

On the morning that you are due to perform a total abdominal hysterectomy with ovarian conservation, your patient says that she now wishes to have a subtotal hysterectomy and bilateral salpingo-oophorectomy (BSO). Explain your counselling and actions.

Examiner's mark sheet

1. The candidate would ask the patient if she is sure that this is what she wants and asks why she has changed her mind.   [1 mark]

2. Explains the pros and cons of total versus subtotal hysterectomy:

    • Pros:

        – removal of the cervix, so there is no need for further smears (provided that histology and previous smears were normal)

        – there is also a lesser risk (negligible risk) of vaginal spotting/ bleeding than after a subtotal hysterectomy.

    • Cons: removal of the cervix will require further dissection of the bladder and the operation may take longer.   [2 marks]

3. Explains the pros and cons of BSO and conservation:

    • Pros:

        – removing the ovaries and tubes removes the background risk of developing ovarian carcinoma (approximately 1 in 70 lifetime risk if no family history) or fallopian tube cancer (extremely rare anyway)

        – it also removes her risk of developing benign ovarian cysts in later life.

- Cons:

    – removal of the ovaries in the vast majority of women of reproductive age will result in the acute onset of menopausal symptoms; this may necessitate the need for hormone replacement therapy (HRT), the pros and cons of which also need to be explained to the patient

    – reassures the patient that there is no real disadvantage in removing the fallopian tubes.   [2 marks]

4.   Counsels her on the pros and cons of using HRT.   [2 marks]

5.   After careful counselling, if the patient were absolutely happy with her new decision, had no further questions and were willing to sign a new updated consent form, then the candidate would be happy to go ahead with a subtotal hysterectomy with BSO that morning. Should there be any doubt in the patient's mind, the operation would be cancelled to allow her more time to consider her options.   [3 marks]

Station 19

Candidate instructions

You are asked to explain, quickly and succinctly, the meaning of the following laboratory test results and how you would manage such patients:

- *CVS direct preparation results: karyotype, trisomy 18*

- *booking haemoglobin electrophoresis: HbSS*

- *booking hepatitis B serology: surface antigen positive.*

Examiner's mark sheet

CVS direct preparation results: karyotype, trisomy 18.

1. The candidate explains that these are preliminary results and that full culture results are likely to be the same in over 99% of cases; however, full culture results may differ from this preliminary result.   [1 mark]

2. Explains that trisomy 18 is Edwards' syndrome, the second most common autosomal trisomy after trisomy 21, and that it is associated with a worse prognosis. Of children born with trisomy 18, 50% die within 2 months and 90% die within the first year of life. They usually suffer from severe learning disabilities, severe congenital malformations such as major heart defects and gastrointestinal anomalies that may be life threatening.   [2 marks]

3. The options of a termination or continuing with the pregnancy, but is non-directive in counselling.   [½ mark]

Booking haemoglobin electrophoresis: HbSS.

1. Explains this is compatible with sickle cell disease as opposed to trait; as such, it is more serious and has a worse prognosis.   [½ mark]

2. The partner's status will need to be tested to determine the probable haemoglobin genotype of the baby; prenatal diagnosis with CVS or amniocentesis can be performed if the patient so wishes.   [1 mark]

3. The need to monitor this pregnancy very closely because of the increased risk of anaemia, sickle crises, IUGR, pre-eclampsia and intrauterine death.   [1 mark]

4.   During pregnancy the candidate would: ensure that the patient is always well hydrated, reduce the risk of infections, limit the degree of anaemia and monitor her continuously during labour with good analgesia – all aimed at reducing the risk of sickle crises. Oxygen therapy, opiate analgesics, antibiotics and intravenous hydration would be used in the event of a crisis.   [1 mark]

Booking hepatitis B serology: surface antigen positive.

1.   This is consistent with a hepatitis B infection at some time, although further information is required on the patient's hepatitis antigen HBeAg (if positive indicates higher infectivity) and hepatitis antibody HBeAb (if positive indicates less infectivity) status.   [1 mark]

2.   The need to know the patient's recent liver function test results and possibly arrange for a liver ultrasound scan.   [½] mark

3.   There is a small risk of vertical transmission to the baby. The candidate would allow vaginal delivery, but would avoid invasive monitoring such as fetal scalp electrodes and fetal blood sampling. Hepatitis B and C infections are not contraindications to breast-feeding.   [1 mark]

4.   Advises immunising the baby with hepatitis B vaccine at birth.

[½ mark]

Station 20

Candidate instructions

You are asked to explain, quickly and succinctly, the meaning of the following laboratory test results and how you would manage such patients:

- *A 29-year-old woman on day 4 of her menstrual cycle has the following blood results: free androgen index 7.9 IU/ml, luteinising hormone (LH) 12.5 mU/ml, follicle-stimulating hormone (FSH) 4.8 mU/ml.*

- *A gynaecological ultrasound report showing a right-sided, partly solid, partly cystic ovarian cyst in a 47-year-old woman.*

- *A cervical smear result: apoptotic and ghost cells consistent with microinvasive disease.*

Examiner's mark sheet

A 29-year-old woman on day 4 of her menstrual cycle has the following blood results: free androgen index 7.9 IU/ml, LH 12.5 mU/ml, FSH 4.8 mU/ml.

1. The biochemical results support a diagnosis of polycystic ovarian syndrome, although this requires confirmation on ultrasonography and the existence of relevant symptoms, including oligomenorrhoea, hirsutism, subfertility, acne and obesity.   [2½ marks]

2. This affects around 15–20% of the female population and, although it may cause no significant symptoms, it may be associated with a risk of diabetes mellitus in later life and a small increased risk of endometrial cancer.   [2½ marks]

3. Treatment would depend on symptomatology.   [1 mark]

A gynaecological ultrasound report showing a right-sided, partly solid, partly cystic ovarian cyst in a 47-year-old woman.

1. The presence of solid and cystic components is suggestive of ovarian malignancy, which must be ruled out.   [1 mark]

2. The candidate would explore her history, in particular how long ago this finding was made, any associated pain, whether or not she is still

menstruating, any family history of ovarian cancer or personal history of endometriosis. [2½ marks]

3. Says that they would like to request tests for tumour markers such as CA-125. [½ mark]

4. Should the cyst have a suspicion of malignancy, the candidate would discuss the findings with a local gynaecological oncologist with regard to surgical management. [2½ marks]

5. Depending on the patient's wishes and analysis of ultrasound and CA-125 results, surgical management could involve: ovarian cystectomy; unilateral oophorectomy with possible biopsy of the other ovary; or total abdominal hysterectomy, BSO and omentectomy. [2½ marks]

Cervical smear result: apoptotic and ghost cells present that are consistent with microinvasive disease.

1. Explains that the patient would be referred for urgent colposcopy (within 2 weeks) and assessment for signs of microinvasion – pollarded vessels, corkscrew vessels, large-volume acetowhite, peeled–rolled edges of acetowhite. [2½ marks]

2. If microinvasion is suspected, colposcopy and excisional biopsy will be sufficient (LLETZ [large loop excision of the transformation zone] or a cone biopsy). [3 marks]

Station 21

Candidate instructions

You are the duty specialist registrar on call when a 36 weeks' pregnant woman who is having convulsions is rushed in by ambulance. Explain your management.

Examiner's mark sheet

1. The candidate would resuscitate the patient: ensuring adequate airway/clearing it if necessary, giving oxygen by face mask, placing the patient in the recovery position in a safe surrounding where she is unlikely to injure herself, and checking maternal pulse, blood pressure and oxygen saturation. The candidate would call for help, including the anaesthetist and consultant obstetrician on call for the labour ward.   [2 marks]

2. Asks for relevant medical history, pre-eclampsia or a history of epilepsy and examines the patient.   [1 mark]

3. The candidate would establish an intravenous access, give magnesium sulphate 4 g in 10 ml 0.9% (physiological) saline slowly over 15 minutes, and set up a maintenance infusion of magnesium sulphate 1 g/h. Would give intravenous antihypertensives, eg hydralazine or labetolol, if appropriate.   [2 marks]

4. Would take blood samples for urgent FBC, U&Es, urate, liver function tests, clotting profile and 'group and serum save'.   [1 mark]

5. If the patient is still fitting after 15 min, the candidate would give a further bolus of magnesium sulphate 2 g in 10 ml 0.9% saline over 15 minutes and seek consultant assistance.   [1 mark]

6. If patient is still fitting, the candidate would give intravenous diazepam 5 mg every 5 minutes for 15 minutes.   [1 mark]

7. In the unlikely event of continued fitting, says that they would consider giving intravenous thiopental.   [1 mark]

8. After the woman's observations and conditions have been stabilised, would possibly deliver the baby by Caesarean section.   [1 mark]

Station 22

Candidate instructions

Mrs Double is 21 weeks into her first pregnancy with twins. She has had no complications in this pregnancy, but would like to discuss the delivery with you. Explain how you would carry out the delivery of her twins.

Examiner's mark sheet

1. The candidate asks whether it is a monochorionic or dichorionic twin pregnancy. [½ mark]

2. Checks for medical, surgical or obstetric problems. [½ mark]

3. Explains that there is still debate about how best to deliver twins, but if first twin is cephalic then aim for vaginal delivery. [1 mark]

4. There is a need for continuous electronic fetal monitoring in labour with a CTG (cardiotocography) and fetal scalp electrode (FSE) if membranes are ruptured. [1 mark]

5. Once in labour involve anaesthetists and paediatricians. [1 mark]

6. After delivering first twin, clamp the cord, monitor the fetal heart. [1 mark]

7. Palpate the mother's abdomen to ensure a longitudinal lie of the second twin; an ultrasound scan may be used for this. Start an oxytocin infusion if contractions are absent and the fetal heart is normal. [1 mark]

8. Perform external cephalic version for a transverse and oblique lie, and allow a vaginal breech delivery of second twin if it is so presenting. [1 mark]

9. Aim for 30-minute inter-twin delivery interval if the CTG is normal. [1 mark]

10. If the presenting part of the second twin is still high, allow descent into the pelvis; provided that there are no concerns for fetal well-being, aim to deliver in theatre/trial of instrumental vaginal delivery or an emergency Caesarean section as appropriate. [1 mark]

11. If there is a significant risk of postpartum haemorrhage (PPH), manage the third stage actively and give oxytocin infusion for 4–6 hours after delivery. [1 mark]

Station 23

Candidate instructions

Your clinical director is concerned that there are inappropriate inductions of labour for postdate pregnancies. You have been asked to audit the number of postdate inductions of labour in your hospital. Explain in detail exactly how you would do this.

Examiner's mark sheet

1. Defines audit. [1 mark]

2. Sets standard – RCOG guidelines recommend induction of labour (IOL) beyond 41 weeks. [1 mark]

3. Understands the rationale for IOL beyond 41+ weeks and not after 43 weeks. [1 mark]

4. Would consult with the clinical director/audit office to determine what other questions/data to analyse. These may include the type and dose of prostaglandin used, artificial rupture of membranes and total dose of oxytocin used. [1 mark]

5. Would determine whether audit has been performed previously and any relevant recommendations from such an audit. [1 mark]

6. The candidate would set time limits, determine specific records for analysis and seek help from the audit department in obtaining notes. [1 mark]

7. Would construct an audit questionnaire to be filled out for each IOL (audit tool) and enter the information obtained into a computer database. [1 mark]

8. Would analyse data and compare findings with the standard. [1 mark]

9. Discusses how a change in practice may be implemented, although local policies and standards may differ from the RCOG guidelines. [1 mark]

10. The candidate would re-audit the IOL process after the change has been instituted to close the loop. [1 mark]

Station 24

Candidate instructions

Mrs Lagard is a 21-year-old French woman in her first pregnancy, and is now 20 weeks' pregnant. She is referred to you with the results of a Toxoplasma blood test performed 2 weeks ago at her request. She has no history of any illness and does not keep cats.

The microbiology laboratory report shows:

- Toxoplasma *IgG positive*

- Toxoplasma *IgM positive.*

She would like to know the significance of the test and what the possible options are for her in this pregnancy.

Examiner's mark sheet

1. The candidate gives a simple explanation of what *Toxoplasma* is (a protozoan) and what the test means (past and recent exposure to or reactivation of *Toxoplasma*). [1 mark]

2. Explains where the infection may have come from (cat litter or cold meats or salads). [1 mark]

3. Although she has recently had *Toxoplasma* infection, it does not mean that her baby will be either infected or affected. [1 mark]

4. The baby is less likely to be infected at earlier gestations, but if infected the consequences are usually more severe, including microcephaly, hydrocephaly, intracranial calcifications and chorioretinitis. [2 marks]

5. Follow-up in the fetal medicine unit to discuss further investigations, such as cordocentesis, to see whether the fetus is infected. The risk of miscarriage with cordocentesis is about 2%. [2 marks]

6. Explains the pros and cons of medical treatment with drugs, eg spiramycin – 50% reduction of transmission with no fetal toxicity. [1 mark]

7. The possibility of follow-up scans to see if there are any signs of infection (microcephaly, hydrocephaly, intracranial calcifications). [1 mark]

8. There is a risk of intrauterine death or major handicap. She should see a paediatrician to discuss the long-term prognosis. [1 mark]

Station 25

Candidate instructions

You are asked to see Mrs Simpson who is a 32-year-old G3 P2 woman because your consultant is away.

She works as a sculptor and lives in a comfortable semi-rural house with her husband and two children.

She has had a normal delivery with her first baby and a Caesarean section for a footling breech in her second pregnancy. Both babies are well and weighed 7 lb 6 oz and 7lb 10 oz, respectively.

She is 36 weeks' gestation, cephalic presentation, appropriate size and with no complications in this pregnancy.

Mrs Simpson is requesting a home delivery and is insistent, despite counselling against home delivery by the midwife.

Role player's instructions

- You are 32 years old, a self-employed sculptor, who lives in a comfortable house with your two children aged 4 and 6 years. You are well educated and informed but not easily persuaded into changing your mind.

- You did not enjoy the experience of a Caesarean section in your second pregnancy, particularly as you do not like taking any medicines or drugs.

- You are insistent, impolite and not open to reasoned debate.

- You would like a home delivery; you would be resistant to transfer to hospital in labour and would like a physiological third stage.

Examiner's mark sheet

1. Polite, respectful, non-judgemental approach (in the face of provocation) but insistent on giving the facts about a trial of scar.

    [2 marks]

2. Information about the scar dehiscence rate of 1 in 200–300 trials of scar. [2 marks]

3. Information about the successful vaginal delivery rate of 65–70%.

    [2 marks]

4. If a home birth is chosen there is a 30–35% chance of an intrapartum transfer to hospital. [1 mark]

5. The absence of electronic monitoring (in a home birth) may delay the diagnosis of scar dehiscence. [1 mark]

6. After discussion of the issues, gives clear unambiguous explanation that the following probably will all add to the risk of a PPH and potential transfer to hospital:

    – the resistance to accept advice on the place of delivery

    – the intention of not accepting the midwife's advice on intrapartum transfer

    – a physiological second stage.

    All could potentially have grave consequences but the decision is the patient's responsibility. [2 marks]

Station 26

Candidate instructions

Mrs Angela Robinson has come to see you for a postnatal visit 6 weeks after a forceps delivery. Her baby is well.

She has some questions about the delivery itself but otherwise there are no issues.

The hospital notes are not available for the consultation.

Role player's instructions

- You have had a forceps delivery for delay in the second stage of labour.

- Since delivery you have been struggling to cope with the baby, whom you describe as a troublesome baby who does not feed or sleep well.

- Your husband works long hours and is unsupportive. You have not resumed sexual intercourse since delivery.

- Your sleep pattern is poor and you are overeating, therefore putting on weight, and this is making you more unhappy.

- Throughout the consultation you are miserable, talk slowly and do not make eye contact with the doctor. You do not say that you are depressed but may reveal that you have a past history of depression.

- You do not have thoughts of suicide or harming the baby.

- You would like to know from the doctor why you needed to be delivered using forceps and was it necessary. Did the forceps delivery make the baby unhappy with you?

Examiner's mark sheet

This is a station where non-verbal clues need to be recognised and the diagnosis of postnatal depression made.

1.   Discussion and explanation that second stage delay is an indication for forceps delivery.   [1 mark]

2.   Evaluation of the patient's physical recovery and health of the baby.
                                                                                          [1 mark]

3.   Recognition of patient's depressed state by gentle questioning of the issues of baby care, family relationships, eating pattern, low mood and sleep disturbance.   [3 marks]

4.   Questioning about ideas of suicide or risk to the baby through either neglect or harm.   [2 marks]

5.   Management plan for referral to GP, community psychiatric nurse (CPN) input or possibly involvement of psychiatrist. All should be explained and discussed sensitively with the patient.   [2 marks]

6.   Reassurance and explanation about the need for therapy, which could involve counselling or/and medication.   [1 mark]

Station 27

Candidate instructions

Mr White is angry that his wife's laparoscopic sterilisation has failed (he already has five children). You are now seeing him in the gynaecology clinic. His wife is ill with morning sickness and could not attend. It is 5 months since you performed the operation and she is now 6 weeks' pregnant. Conduct an interview with Mr White.

Role player's instructions

Be aggressive and very upset at the failure of the sterilisation.
The following are suggested questions/comments for the role player to ask/ say to the candidate:

- Why did this happen?

- How many have you done? Why didn't a more senior doctor do the operation?

- I wasn't told that this could happen, I'm going to sue you.

- I'm going to the newspapers and television.

- I'll report you to the General Medical Council (GMC) and get you struck off.

Threaten the candidate with violence.
Shout and raise your voice:

- Your colleagues who were assisting you were negligent as well, weren't they?

- I want compensation – how much is it worth?

- Why wasn't I given an information leaflet on this before the procedure?

- What are you going to do about it now?

- I'm not satisfied with your explanation, you don't know what you're talking about!

Examiner's mark sheet

Award marks for those candidates who display the following qualities and explain the following points:

1. Is firm, but non-aggressive, with an open posture and does not allow himself or herself to be bullied.   [1 mark]

2. Explains, using non-medical jargon, what happened and why (if possible).   [1 mark]

3. Says it is the patient's right if he wants to take things further, and advises him that the next step would be to contact the chief executive of the trust and the complaints officer.   [1 mark]

4. Tells the complainant that he can go to the papers/TV or seek legal advice or contact the GMC if he wishes.   [1 mark]

5. When Mr White starts shouting, the candidate stays calm, has an open posture, does not argue, says that they can empathise with his predicament – offers the correct lines of contact if he is not satisfied with the explanation.   [1 mark]

6. Does not implicate colleagues, even if the candidate thinks that they are to blame – explains that it is for an independent review panel to decide.   [1 mark]

7. Does not give any cash figures for what compensation Mr and Mrs White are entitled to, if any. Says that it is for the courts to decide, if indeed liability is proven.   [2 marks]

8. Says that it is left to the discretion of the individual doctor obtaining the consent whether the patient needs or requires additional information.   [1 mark]

9. Briefly explains the complaints procedure.   [1 mark]

Station 28

Candidate instructions

You are given a Ventouse cup and a mannequin of a baby in a mother's pelvis, and asked the following questions:

- *Explain the indications for using a Ventouse cup.*
- *Explain what prerequisites have to be satisfied before using a Ventouse cup.*
- *Explain when you would use forceps in preference to a Ventouse cup.*
- *Explain the possible maternal and fetal complications of the Ventouse cup.*
- *Explain which vacuum device you would choose and when you would use it.*
- *Explain what you would do if the cup detached.*
- *Explain whether you would convert to using forceps if the baby were not delivered after three pulls with the Ventouse cup.*

Examiner's mark sheet

1. Explain the indications for using a Ventouse cup: fetal or maternal distress or delay during the second stage of labour.   [1 mark]

2. Explain what prerequisites have to be satisfied before using a Ventouse cup: ideally, the cervix should be fully dilated, with no more than a fifth of the fetal head palpable per abdomen, membranes should be ruptured, the presentation should be cephalic, the maternal bladder empty and the presenting part should be at the level of the spines or below.   [2 marks]

3. Explain when you would use forceps in preference to a Ventouse cup: the Ventouse cup and similar vacuum instruments are often considered the first choice for assisted vaginal delivery over forceps because they are associated with less maternal trauma. If there is a large caput, poor maternal effort, inefficient suction pressure or the gestational age of the fetus is < 34 weeks, forceps should be considered.   [1 mark]

4.   Explain the possible maternal and fetal complications of a Ventouse cup:

– maternal: trauma to the bladder, urethra, uterus, cervix, vagina and haemorrhage

– fetal: scalp trauma/laceration, but rarely necrosis; cephalohaematoma, anaemia, jaundice, subgaleal haemorrhage, alopecia in infancy and retinal haemorrhage.   [1 mark]

5.   Explain which vacuum device you would choose and when you would use it:

– silastic/soft cup would be used for a flexed, synclitic head in an occipitoanterior position

– Malmström for occipitoanterior/transverse positions

– Bird for occiput posterior positions

– kiwi cup for occipitoanterior/transverse/posterior positions.[2 marks]

6.   Explain what you would do if the cup detached: explains that they would consider why it detached. Cites as reasons incorrect placement of the cup, incorrect axis of traction, poor suction pressure, large caput, head too high. Says that, if descent occurred with the pull, they would consider reattaching the cup, but not more than twice and provided that there had been progressive and adequate descent of the fetal head. Explains that delivery may also be completed with a pair of forceps if descent and rotation had been achieved with the Ventouse cup.   [2 marks]

7.   Would you convert to using the forceps if the delivery is not accomplished after three pulls with the Ventouse? Explains that they would not routinely use two different instruments to deliver the baby. However, if the baby's head had descended very low in the pelvis and was in a favourable position, especially where adequate suction pressure was not achievable, or there was poor maternal effort or poor contractions, the delivery could be completed with forceps. A Caesarean section at full dilatation with the head very low in the pelvis may cause more complications than forceps.   [1 mark]

Station 29

Candidate instructions

You are asked to explain the pros and cons of HRT to this role-play patient. She has been referred by her GP to see you in the outpatient department.

Role player's instructions

- You are a 47-year-old married woman who has not had a period for 10 months.

- You have hot flushes and night sweats.

- You are undecided whether or not you want to go on HRT.

- You tend to go to the toilet more frequently than you used to (around 10 times a day), sometimes don't make it in time and occasionally leak urine when you cough or sneeze. You wonder whether HRT may help with your urinary symptoms.

- You have had an appendicectomy.

- You are not taking any medications.

- You smoke 10 cigarettes a day, and have the occasional alcoholic drink.

- Your mother died from breast cancer.

- Please ask the candidate the following questions:

    – Am I menopausal?

    – Will HRT improve my symptoms?

    – Will I get breast cancer?

    – Should I take HRT, and if so which route would you advise and how long should I take it for?

Examiner's mark sheet

1.   The candidate introduces himself or herself, maintains eye contact and listens to the patient.   [½ mark]

2.   Takes an appropriate history: menstrual history, any postcoital
     bleeding, date of her last smear, method of contraception, medical
     history, including risk factors for cardiovascular disease or
     osteoporosis, family history of deep vein thrombosis (DVT) or breast
     or endometrial cancer, and social history, including smoking, alcohol
     and recreational drugs.   [2 marks]

3.   The absence of periods for 1 year without pregnancy, with the
     range of symptoms that the patient currently has, would suggest
     the menopause. Strictly speaking, however, she is in the climacteric
     phase.   [1 mark]

4.   HRT may help to reduce her hot flushes, night sweats and
     possibly urinary urgency, although it will not reverse urinary stress
     incontinence.   [½ mark]

5.   The risk of breast cancer is increased by taking HRT (from 45/1000
     to 90/1000) and more in women with first-degree relatives affected by
     breast cancer.   [1 mark]

6.   The decision to take HRT is entirely that of the patient, although there
     are well-documented advantages and risks including:

     – advantages: reduction in the risks of osteoporosis, colon cancer and
     Alzheimer's disease, aches and pains; improvement of moods, skin,
     hair and teeth

     – risks: an increase in the risk of DVT from 10/100 000 to 30/100 000
     and of breast cancer after 8 years of use, and an increased risk of
     stroke and cardiovascular disease with certain continuous combined
     oral preparations; the candidate explains that they cannot be certain
     whether such risks are present with oestrogen-only therapy. [2 marks]

7.   HRT can be administered orally, or via a skin patch, gel, vaginal route,
     nasal spray or subcutaneous implant.   [1 mark]

8.   Alternatives to HRT: stop smoking, good exercise, and use of calcium
     supplements and bisphosphates.   [1 mark]

9.   SERMs (selective oestrogen receptor modulator) can be used but has
     risks of venous thromboembolism (VTE).   [1 mark]

Station 30

Candidate instructions

You are the specialist registrar on call and have been asked to see Mrs Smith, who is 40 weeks' pregnant and has not felt the baby move today. The sonographer, who cannot see a fetal heart motion on scan, has diagnosed an intrauterine death, and called you to explain the scan findings to Mrs Smith. How would you counsel Mrs Smith?

Role player's instructions

- You are a 28-year-old woman in your first pregnancy.

- This pregnancy was uneventful until today when you haven't felt your baby move.

- You are absolutely distraught at what has happened. You cry repeatedly and ask why this has happened.

- You ask what the next step is. Do I need a Caesarean section now?

- Ask why the baby has died.

- Ask if this will happen again.

Examiner's mark sheet

1. The candidate introduces himself or herself, makes good eye contact, comforts the patient appropriately, asks if her husband is coming and if there is anyone else whom she would like to be contacted, and is able to break the news to the patient and express sympathy. [2 marks]

2. No obvious cause for what has happened, blood for tests, postmortem examination, parents' consent. [2 marks]

3. Discusses the induction process with prostaglandins and explains that a Caesarean section is generally not recommended because it is more risky to the mother's health. [2 marks]

4. Offers the services of a religious representative of her faith, if appropriate, and the phone number of a counsellor and support groups. [1 mark]

5. It is routine practice to obtain a picture of the baby and footprints, which will be kept in the notes, and which she and her husband can view at a later date if they so wish. [1 mark]

6. Discusses her next pregnancy, because it is unlikely that there will be any problems in any future pregnancies; arranges 6-week follow-up appointment with the consultant to review all the results of the investigations. [2 marks]

Abbreviations

ACE	angiotensin-converting enzyme
ACTH	adrenocorticotrophic hormone
AFP	α-fetoprotein
AIDS	acquired immunodeficiency disease syndrome
AIS	adenocarcinoma in situ
ALT	alanine transaminase
AZf	azidothymidine
BMI	body mass index
BP	blood pressure
BPD	biparietal diameter
BPP	biophysical profiles
BRCA	breast cancer
BSO	bilateral salpingo-oophorectomy
CA-125	carcinoembryonic antigen 125
CGIN	cervical glandular intraepithelial neoplasia
CIN	cervical intraepithelial neoplasia
CLASP	Collaborative Low-dose Aspirin
CMV	cytomegalovirus
CNS	central nervous system
COCP	combined oral contraceptive pill
CPA	cyproterone acetate
CPN	community psychiatric nurse
CRL	crown-rump length
CT	computed tomography
CTG	cardiotocography
CVP	central venous pressure
CVS	chorionic villus sampling
CVT	cerebral vein thrombosis
D&C	dilatation and curettage
DHEAS	dehydroepiandrosterone sulphate
DIC	disseminated intravascular coagulation
ECG	electrocardiogram
EEG	electroencephalogram
EFW	estimated fetal weight
EMG	electromyogram
EUA	examination under anaesthesia
FAS	fetal anatomy scan
FBC	full blood count
FBV	fetal blood volume
FDP	fibrin degradation product

FFP	fresh-frozen plasma
FSE	fetal scalp electrode
FSH	follicle-stimulating hormone
GMC	General Medical Council
GnRH	gonadotrophin-releasing hormone
GP	general practitioner
HAART	highly active antiretroviral therapy
Hb	haemoglobin
HbSS	sickle cell anaemia
hCG	human chorionic gonadotrophin
HDU	high-dependency unit
HELLP	haemolysis/elevated liver enzymes/low platelet count
HIA	haemagglutinin inhibition assay
HIV	human immunodeficiency virus
hMG	human menopausal gonadotrophin
HPV	human papilloma virus
HRT	hormone replacement therapy
ICSI	intracytoplasmic sperm injection
IMB	intermenstrual bleeding
INR	international normalised ratio
IOL	induction of labour
ITP	idiopathic thrombocytopenic purpura
ITU	intensive therapy unit
IUCO	intrauterine contraceptive device
IUO	intrauterine device
IUGR	intrauterine growth retardation/restriction
IUI	intrauterine insemination
IUS	Intra-uterine system
IVF	in vitro fertilisation
LAVH	laparoscopically assisted vaginal hysterectomy
LFT	liver function test
LH	luteinising hormone
LLETZ	large loop excision of the transformation zone
LMWH	low-molecular-weight heparin
LSCS	lower segment Caesarean section
MAC-RIA	membrane attack complex radioimmunoassay
MCS	microscopy, culture and sensitivity
MRC	Medical Research Council
MRI	magnetic resonance imaging
MSU	mid-stream urine sample
MTCT	mother-to-child transmission
NHS	National Health Service
NICE	National Institute for Clinical Excellence

NT	nuchal translucency
OC	oral contraceptive
OHSS	ovarian hyperstimulation syndrome
PCOO	polycystic ovary disease
PCOS	polycystic ovary syndrome
PCR	polymerase chain reaction
POS	polydioxanone suture
PET	pre-eclampsia toxaemia
PhCG	progesterone and β human chorionic gonadotrophin
PIO	pelvic inflammatory disease
PMS	urea and electrolytes
PPH	post partum haemorrhage
PPROM	premature prelabour rupture of membranes
PRL	prolactin
RCOG	Royal College of Obstetrics and Gynaecology
RCT	randomised controlled trial
Rh	rhesus
SERM	selective oestrogen receptor modulator
SGA	small-for-gestational age
SHBG	sex hormone-binding globulin
SHO	senior house officer
SLE	systemic lupus erythematosus
STI	sexually transmitted infection
TACE	tumour necrosis factor α converting enzyme
T AH	total abdominal hysterectomy
TEO	thromboembolism disease
TFT	thyroid function test
TOP	termination of pregnancy
TORCH	toxoplasmosis, rubella, cytomegalovirus and herpes
TSH	thyroid-stimulating hormone
TIP	thrombocytopenic purpura
TVS	transvaginal ultrasound
U&Es	urea and electrolytes
USS	ultrasound scan
UTI	urinary tract infection
VALUE	Valsartan antihypertensive long-term use evaluation
VCUG	video-cystourethrography
VH	vaginal hysterectomy
VIN	vaginal intraepithelial neoplasia
VTE	venous thromboembolism

Bibliography

Cochrane Library www.cochrane.org

Edmonds D.K, *Dewhurst's Textbook of Obstetrics and Gynaecology for Postgraduates*, Sixth Edition, Blackwell Science, 1999

Nelson-Piercy C, *Handbook of Obstetric Medicine*, ISIS Medical Media, 2000

Royal College of Obstetricians & Gynaecologists, *The Green Top Guidelines*, RCOG Press www.rcog.org.uk

Shafi M, Luesley D, Jordan J, *Handbook of Gynaecological Oncology*, Churchill Livingstone, 2001

The Obstetrician & Gynaecologist, RCOG Press, 2001-6 www.rcog.org.uk/togonline

Index

abortion *see* miscarriage; termination of
pregnancy
abruptio placenta 169
addiction 182–3
adverse effects *see* side effects
age, care of older mothers 150–1
alcohol abuse 42, 85, 170–1
α-fetoprotein (AFP) 43, 86
5α-reductase deficiency 36, 81
amenorrhoea
    premature ovarian failure 25, 75
    primary 6, 63
    secondary 192–3
amniocentesis 52, 92
amniotic fluid 18, 69
    embolism 169
    oligohydramnios 158–9
anaesthetics in labour 50, 91
anal sphincter injury 23, 24, 73, 74
aneuploidy
    Down syndrome 56, 95, 186–7
    Edwards syndrome 210
    'soft' markers 12, 66
    Turner syndrome 29, 77
angry relatives, dealing with 226–7
antibiotics, audit of use 184–5
anti-D prophylaxis 16, 68
antidepressants 125
antiphospholipid syndrome 135
Apgar score 52, 92
appendicitis 56, 95
aspirin 135, 155
assisted reproduction
    clomifene citrate 27, 76
    complications (general) 4, 27, 61, 76
    consultation for 196–7
    OHSS 27, 76, 128–9
assisted vaginal delivery 152–3, 228–9
audit procedures
    induction of labour 218–19
    prophylactic antibiotic use 184–5
azidothymidine (AZT) 147
azoospermia 26, 75

bacterial vaginosis 9, 65
bad news, counselling 232–3
βhCG (β human chorionic
    gonadotrophin) 38, 83
bilateral salpingo-oophorectomy (BSO)
    123, 208–9
bladder
    detrusor overactivity 6, 62
    innervation 37, 82
    intraoperative complications 7, 63
    physiology 5, 62
    stress incontinence 24–5, 74
breech presentation 175

caesarean section
    complications 37, 82, 156–7
    emergency 153, 160–1
    vaginal delivery after 222–3
cancer
    toxicity of chemotherapy 35, 81
    see also specific sites
candidiasis 3, 61
cardiovascular system
    peripartum cardiomyopathy 14, 67
    in pregnancy 12, 45, 66, 88
    prosthetic valves 16, 68
cervical cancer
    epidemiology 139
    invasive 8, 64
    pre-invasive 32–3, 79
    risk factors 32, 79
    smear tests 23, 73, 139, 213
    staging 8, 64
cervical glandular intraepithelial
    neoplasia (CGIN) 33, 79
cervical incompetence

cerclage for 162–3
cervical length 47, 89
cervical intraepithelial neoplasia (CIN)
  32, 79
chemotherapy, side effects 35, 81
chickenpox 17, 69
childbirth
  anaesthetic use 50, 91
  audit of induction of labour 218–19
  breech presentation 175
  caesarean section 156–7, 160–1
  delay in second stage of labour
    152–3
  face presentation 44, 87
  home delivery 222–3
  management (general) 15, 68
  tocolysis 12, 66
  twins 216–17
  Ventouse delivery 228–9
cholestasis, obstetric 41, 85, 166–7
chorionic villus sampling (CVS) 210
chromosomal abnormalities
  Down syndrome 56, 95, 186–7
  Edwards syndrome 210
  recurrent miscarriage 135
  'soft' markers 12, 66
  Turner syndrome 29, 77
cleft lip/palate 13, 67
clomifene citrate 27, 76, 129
CMV (cytomegalovirus) 44, 55, 87, 94
coagulation in pregnancy
  clotting factors 57, 95
  DIC 168–9
  thromboprophylaxis 154–5, 180–1
colposcopy 111
complaints procedures 226–7
congenital adrenal hyperplasia 6, 28,
  63, 76
congenital infections
  asymptomatic bacteriuria 53, 93
  chickenpox 17, 69
  CMV 44, 55, 87, 94
  listeriosis 55, 94

parvovirus B19 55, 94
rubella 53, 93, 198–9
toxoplasmosis 54, 94, 220–1
contraception
  consultations for 178–9, 202–3
  copper coil 4, 61
  emergency 3, 4–5, 61, 62, 178–9
  Mirena coil 120–1
  progesterone-only pill 30, 78
  stopping 7, 64
convulsions 148–9, 214–15
CVS (chorionic villus sampling) 210
cyproterone acetate (CPA) 113
cytomegalovirus (CMV) 44, 55, 87, 94

danazol 39, 83, 123
depression 224–5
detrusor function 5, 6, 62
dextran 155
diabetes mellitus
  management of convulsions 149
  pre-pregnancy clinics 143
  type 1 in pregnancy 51, 91–2, 204–5
diagnostic tests see prenatal screening;
  screening tests
diathermy 200–1
diethylstilbestrol 34, 80
disseminated intravascular coagulation
  (DIC) 168–9
domestic violence 176–7
Doppler ultrasonography
  umbilical artery 47, 88, 159
  uteroplacental 54, 93
Down syndrome 56, 95, 186–7
drugs of abuse 182–3
dyspareunia 13, 67

eclampsia 149
ectopic pregnancy 6, 38, 63, 83
Edwards syndrome (trisomy 18) 210
electrocardiography in pregnancy 45, 88
emergency contraception 3, 61, 178–9
  copper IUCDs 4, 61

progesterone-only 5, 62
encephalocele 46, 88
endometrial cancer 39, 84, 139
endometrial hyperplasia 33, 80, 121
endometrioid carcinoma of the ovary
    10, 65
endometriosis 38, 83
    treatment 39, 83–4, 122–3
epidemiology
    gynaecological cancers 138–9
    HIV infection 11, 66
epidural anaesthesia 50, 91
essay-writing technique 100–3
estradiol 129

face presentation 44, 87
faecal incontinence 23–4, 73–4
fatty liver 164–5
fetal alcohol syndrome 42, 85, 170–1
fetal anaemia 18, 69
fetal assessment 46, 88
fetal circulation 42, 86
fetal death
    counselling 232–3
    DIC and 169
    of one twin 20, 71
fetal hormones 48, 89
fetal hydrops 18, 57, 69, 96
fetal screening see prenatal screening
fetal size, SGA 17, 69
fibroids 108–9
fistulas 48, 89
fits 148–9, 214–15
fluid balance 137
forceps delivery 229
fungal infections 3, 61

galactorrhoea 192–3
genetic counselling 135, 143
genetic diseases 45, 87
    see also chromosomal abnormalities
germ-cell tumours 35, 81
gestrinone 39, 84

gonadotrophin-releasing hormone
    (GnRH) analogues 28, 76, 109, 123
gonadotrophins
    in assisted reproduction 129
    in disease states 31, 79
gonorrhoea 10, 65
grand-multiparity 150–1

haemodynamic changes in pregnancy
    15, 68
haemoglobinopathy 13, 66, 210–11
haemorrhage
    DIC and 169
    during caesarean sections 157
    ovarian cysts 26, 75
    perforated uterus 130–1
    postpartum 19, 70, 194–5
    see also intermenstrual bleeding
haemostasis, diathermy for 200–1
heart see cardiovascular system
HELLP syndrome 52, 92, 169
heparin 135, 155
hepatitis B 211
hereditary diseases 45, 87
heroin addiction 182–3
herpes gestationis 19, 70
hirsutism 30, 78, 112–13
HIV
    assisted reproduction and 196–7
    epidemiology 11, 66
    in pregnancy 20, 70, 146–7
home delivery 222–3
hormone replacement therapy (HRT)
    230–1
human papilloma viruses (HPVs) 32, 79
hydatidiform mole 7, 10, 63, 65
hydrops fetalis 18, 57, 69, 96
hyperemesis gravidarum 50, 90, 136–7
hyperprolactinaemia 29, 31, 77, 78
hypertension in pregnancy 49, 90, 190–1
    HELLP syndrome 52, 92, 169
    pre-eclampsia 49, 90
hyperthyroidism 47, 89

hypothyroidism 47, 89
hysterectomy
    antibiotic use 184–5
    counselling of alternatives 208–9
    for endometriosis 123
    laparoscopically assisted 126–7
    for menorrhagia 115
hysterosalpingography 133
hysteroscopy 111

idiopathic thrombocytopenic purpura
    (ITP) 42, 85
in vitro fertilisation (IVF) *see* assisted
    reproduction
incontinence *see* faecal *or* urinary
    incontinence
infertility
    azoospermia 26, 75
    premature ovarian failure 25, 75
    primary amenorrhoea 6, 63
    recurrent miscarriage 29, 77, 134–5
    see also assisted reproduction
inflammatory bowel disease 50, 91
inheritance patterns 45, 87
instrumental delivery 152–3, 228–9
intermenstrual bleeding 110–11
intrauterine contraceptive devices
    (IUCDs)
    copper 4, 61
    Mirena coil 3, 61, 120–1
intrauterine death
    counselling 232–3
    DIC and 169
    of one twin 20, 71
intrauterine growth restriction (IUGR)
    diagnosis 159
    management 140–1
    SGA fetus 17, 69
iron supplementation 45, 87
ITP (idiopathic thrombocytopenic
    purpura) 42, 85
IUCDs *see* intrauterine contraceptive
    devices

IUGR *see* intrauterine growth restriction
IVF *see* assisted reproduction

jaundice, neonatal 43, 86

kidney failure in pregnancy 144–5
Krukenberg's tumours 35, 80

labour *see* childbirth
laparoscopically assisted vaginal
    hysterectomy (LAVH) 115, 126–7
laparoscopy 7, 63, 127
leiomyosarcoma 11, 66
levonorgestrel intrauterine system
    (Mirena coil) 3, 61, 120–1
listeriosis 55, 94
liver disease
    fatty liver 165–6
    hepatitis B 211
    neonatal jaundice 43, 86
    obstetric cholestasis 41, 85, 166–7
LMWH (low molecular weight heparin)
    155, 181

magnetic resonance imaging (MRI) 133
maternal age, advanced 150–1
menopause
    HRT 230–1
    management of symptoms 124–5
    metabolic changes 28, 77
menorrhagia 114–15, 121
Mirena coil 3, 61, 120–1
miscarriage
    recurrent 29, 77, 134–5
    second trimester 162–3
MRCOG Part 2 examination
    essay-writing technique 100–3
    structure ix, 99
    syllabus ix–xii
MRI (magnetic resonance imaging) 133
multiparity 150–1
myomectomy 109

negative predictive value 21, 71
Neisseria gonorrhoeae 10, 65
neonates
    Apgar score 52, 92
    jaundice 43, 86
neural tube defects 46, 88, 188–9
neurology of the urinary tract 37, 82
nuchal translucency 186–7, 206–7

oestrogens 125, 129
OHSS (ovarian hyperstimulation
    syndrome) 27, 76, 128–9
oligohydramnios 18, 69, 158–9
oral contraception
    combined pill 7, 64
    for gynaecological disorders 113,
    123
    progesterone-only pill 30, 78
osteoporosis 31, 78
ovarian cancer 9, 64
    borderline 11, 65
    cell types 35, 81
    diagnosis and management 212–13
    endometrioid 10, 65
    epidemiology 139
    metastatic (Krukenberg's) 35, 80
    serous cystadenocarcinoma 36, 81
    torsion and 26, 75
ovarian cysts 38, 83, 212–13
    haemorrhage and 26, 75
ovarian failure, premature 25, 75
ovarian hyperstimulation syndrome
    (OHSS) 27, 76, 128–9
ovarian torsion 26, 75

pancreatitis 56, 95
parturition *see* childbirth
parvovirus B19 55, 94
peripartum cardiomyopathy 14, 67
peritoneum, postoperative closure 37,
    82
placenta
    adherence 41, 85

premature detachment 169
polycystic ovarian syndrome 112–13,
    212
polyhydramnios 18, 69
positive predictive value 21, 71
postnatal depression 224–5
postpartum haemorrhage (PPH) 19, 70,
    194–5
pre-eclampsia
    aetiology 49, 90
    consultation for 190–1
    HELLP syndrome 52, 92, 169
premature labour, tocolysis for 12, 66
premature ovarian failure 25, 75
prenatal screening
    AFP 43, 86
    amniocentesis 52, 92
    counselling 186–9, 206–7, 210
    CVS 210
    Down syndrome in twin pregnancies
    186–7
    nuchal translucency 186–7, 206–7
    second trimester 43, 86
    spina bifida 188–9
    ultrasonography 12, 54, 66, 93, 141,
    159, 186–9
pre-pregnancy clinics 142–3
presentation
    breech 175
    face 44, 87
    occipitotransverse 153
progesterone
    in ectopic pregnancy 38, 83
    in emergency contraception 5, 62
    for endometriosis 123
    for menopausal symptoms 125
    progesterone-only pill 30, 78
prolactin
    hyperprolactinaemia 29, 31, 77, 78
    prolactinoma 192–3
pruritis *see* cholestasis, obstetric
pseudohermaphroditism (5α-reductase
    deficiency) 36, 81

puberty, precocious 30, 78

radiology, diagnostic 132–3
rectovaginal fistulas 48, 89
renal failure in pregnancy 144–5
rhesus disease
    anti-D prophylaxis 16, 68
    fetal anaemia 18, 69
rheumatoid arthritis 14, 67
rubella 53, 93, 198–9

screening tests
    for cancers 23, 73, 139
    statistics 21, 71
    see also prenatal screening
seizures 148–9, 214–15
sensitivity 21, 71
septicaemia 169
sexually transmitted infections 10, 65
shoulder dystocia 48, 90
sickle cell disease 13, 66, 210–11
side effects
    anti-cancer drugs 35, 81
    hyperprolactinaemia 31, 78
small-for-gestational-age (SGA) 17, 69
    see also intrauterine growth
    restriction
smoking in pregnancy 51, 91
specificity 21, 71
spina bifida 188–9
statistics
    distribution 21, 71
    screening tests 21, 71
streptococcal infections 13, 66
stress incontinence 24–5, 74
substance abuse
    alcohol 42, 85, 170–1
    heroin 182–3
surgery
    caesarean section 153, 156–7,
    160–1
    cervical cerclage 162–3
    complications 7, 63, 156–7

diathermy 200–1
for endometriosis 123
for fibroids 109
hysterectomy 115, 123, 126–7,
184–5, 208–9
for menorrhagia 115
peritoneal closure 37, 82
for stress incontinence 25, 74
for vulval cancer 118–19
wound dehiscence 36, 82
systemic lupus erythematosus (SLE)
14, 67

TAH (total abdominal hysterectomy)
115, 123, 208–9
teratogens
antiepileptics 13, 67
diethylstilbestrol 34, 80
warfarin 155
termination of pregnancy
complications 130–1
failure of 4, 61
testosterone 125
thalassaemia 13, 66
thromboprophylaxis 154–5, 180–1
thyroid disease 47, 89
tibolone 125
tocolysis 12, 66
total abdominal hysterectomy (TAH)
115, 123, 208–9
toxicity of chemotherapy 35, 81
toxoplasmosis 54, 94, 220–1
trisomy 18 (Edwards syndrome)
210
trisomy 21 (Down syndrome) 56, 95,
186–7
trophoblastic disease 7, 10, 63, 65
Turner syndrome 29, 77
twin pregnancies
death of one twin 20, 71
delivery 216–17
monochorionic diamniotic 53, 92,
186–7

prenatal testing for Down syndrome 186–7

ultrasonography
in assisted reproduction 129
for gynaecological disorders 111, 133
in pregnancy 54, 93
cervical length measurement 47, 89
Doppler 47, 54, 88, 93, 159
nuchal translucency 186–7, 206–7
'soft' markers of aneuploidy 12, 66
spina bifida 188–9
umbilical artery scanning 47, 88, 159
ureter 37, 82
urinary incontinence
detrusor overactivity 6, 62
diagnosis 116–17
stress incontinence 24–5, 74
urinary tract
anatomy 37, 82
bladder physiology 5, 62
infections 5, 53, 62, 93
intraoperative complications 7, 63
uterine artery
Doppler ultrasonography 54, 93
embolisation 109
uterus
endometrial cancer 39, 84, 139
endometrial hyperplasia 33, 80, 121
fibroid management 108–9
leiomyosarcoma 11, 66
perforated 130–1
see also hysterectomy

vacuum cups 228–9
vaginal bleeding
intermenstrual 110–11
PPH 19, 70, 194–5
vaginal cancer 139
vaginal delivery
after caesarean section 222–3
assisted 152–3, 228–9
breech presentation 175
vaginal infections
bacterial vaginosis 9, 65
candidiasis 3, 61
vaginal intraepithelial neoplasia (VIN) 33, 79
varicella 17, 69
venography 133
ventilation–perfusion scans 133
Ventouse delivery 228–9
vesicovaginal fistulas 48, 89
vomiting 50, 90, 136–7
vulval cancer 34, 80
epidemiology 139
prevention of postoperative morbidity 118–19
treatment 34, 80
vulvovaginal candidiasis 3, 61

warfarin 143, 155, 181
wound dehiscence 36, 82

X rays 133
XO (Turner) syndrome 29, 77

zidovudine 147